PHANTOM
PLAGUE

PHANTOM PLAGUE

HOW TUBERCULOSIS SHAPED HISTORY

VIDYA KRISHNAN

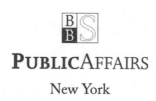

PUBLICAFFAIRS

New York

PublicAffairs
Hachette Book Group
1290 Avenue of the Americas, New York, NY 10104
www.publicaffairsbooks.com
@Public_Affairs

Printed in the United States of America

First Edition: February 2022

Published by PublicAffairs, an imprint of Perseus Books, LLC, a subsidiary of Hachette Book Group, Inc. The PublicAffairs name and logo is a trademark of the Hachette Book Group.

The Hachette Speakers Bureau provides a wide range of authors for speaking events. To find out more, go to www.hachettespeakersbureau.com or call (866) 376-6591.

The publisher is not responsible for websites (or their content) that are not owned by the publisher.

Library of Congress Control Number: 2021949372

ISBNs: 9781541768468 (hardcover), 9781541768475 (e-book)

LSC-C

Printing 1, 2021

To the fallen.

Every year, 10.4 million new cases of tuberculosis are reported globally, and nearly one-third of the world's population has latent TB, a dormant version of this ancient disease. Nearly 2.8 million of the afflicted —more than anywhere else in the world—live in India.

This book is dedicated to the memory of all those who died of tuberculosis. Singled out for special remembrance is Shreya Tripathi, whose life inspired this book.

CONTENTS

PHANTOM
PLAGUE

INTRODUCTION

After a steady decline throughout most of the twentieth century, tuberculosis is back with a ferocity never experienced by humanity before. A world we thought we had left behind—one in which a pathogen could wipe out entire families as doctors helplessly watched—is once again ahead of us.

In a world where quarantines, travel bans, and lockdowns are normalized, the rise of antibiotic-resistant bacteria is an urgent global threat. The indiscriminate consumption of antibiotics during the pandemic (ivermectin, dexamethasone, hydroxychloroquine, favipiravir, azithromycin, etc.) has reached a whole new level of abuse, something that is sure to cast a long shadow on global health.

Superbugs, created by overuse and misuse of antibiotics, have brought the postantibiotic era one step closer. In the nineteenth century, before we had antibiotics, a simple cut or wound could kill us. Antibiotics changed that. Working under the illusion that antibiotics were essential for every sneeze and cold, we have collectively overused antibiotics to the point that they have become ineffective. We are now returning to a time when a simple cut to your finger could leave you fighting for your life.

The most basic operations—getting an appendix removed or having a hip replacement—could become deadly. Childbirth could once again become frequently fatal for young women.

In 2015, BBC ran an analysis under the headline "Antibiotic Apocalypse" in which the World Health Organization warned that "many common infections will no longer have a cure and, once again, could kill unabated."[1] The US Centers for Disease Control pointed to the emergence of "nightmare bacteria," and the chief medical officer for England, Dame Sally Davies, has evoked parallels with the "apocalypse."

The drug-resistant avatar of tuberculosis is a plague worthy of the twenty-first century.

While it is perceived to be a disease of the past in the West, one cannot go a day without coming across tuberculosis in the East. Although TB is curable, in the "clinical deserts," it has found a way to stage a frightening comeback. While the bacteria constantly mutate, humans have remained prisoners to their biases—race, caste, and class—depleting our capacity to keep pace with this evolving foe.

This book tells the story of the global battle against tuberculosis, which will be won, or more likely lost, in India, the world's largest consumer of antibiotics. India has had an antibiotic policy since 2011, but regulation has not made any dent on irrational use of these medicines. For the public, the threat of antibiotic resistance is vague and in the future, while the advantages of self-medicating, in a health system known for its inaccessibility, are immediate.

Diseases, much like individuals, cannot exist in isolation.

They have ancestry and exert significant influence on societies. An appreciation of their history is central to altering the outcome of a "war" we are in serious danger of losing. This biography of the bacteria aims to demystify it by going back to its origin story before bringing its current iteration into focus.

Like all great plagues, tuberculosis has irrevocably changed the fabric of human society. The sheer scale of human suffering it has inflicted has inspired great art, literature, poetry, and operatic tragedies. It has also inspired magical thinking, xenophobia, and science denialism. This book is not about medicine or science or history alone. It is about the interplay of these things.

Tuberculosis demonstrates what happens to science when it leaves the lab setting and interacts with flawed human beings: patients, doctors, politicians, and rabble-rousers, all of whom have a unique effect on the course of the plague. The pathogen reveals as much about us, its hosts, as we have been able to uncover about the pathogen—hence this exploration of vampires, Victorian-era fashion, India's original sin, great wars, flawed heroes, and many patently villainous as well as joyously selfless people.

Two central questions drive the narrative: How did we get to where we are? Where do we go from here?

I have spent the last decade reporting on how drug-resistant (DR) TB has devastated families in one of the world's most overcrowded megacities, Mumbai, India's financial engine. The development of the mutant strains of the bacteria in a rich, cosmopolitan city is a glimpse of the postantibiotic era dawning on all of us.

The story of TB also demonstrates that we can no longer discuss modern medicine—the fruits of which have been withheld from the vast majority of humanity—without discussing race, class, and caste.

This book is an attempt to place the global tuberculosis pandemic in the context of the racial politics of our times.

Global health policies, officially color blind, have left our health to the whims of a handful of pharmaceutical corporations, philanthropists, and politicians. Consequently, a century's worth of medical progress has not been able to stop viral and bacterial disasters, which are becoming more and more difficult to contain. As I was working on this book, the world had been brought to its knees by wave after wave of coronavirus infections. Despite that, and despite the heroic efforts of battle-scarred veterans who fought for affordable drug pricing, by May 2021, only 1 percent of the 1.3 billion vaccines injected around the world had been administered in Africa.

Nearly 216.3 million people have contracted the disease, while the deaths have surged to more than 4.5 million by September 2021.

The immensity of the global pandemic has not been able to override a global health order in which the white medical establishment treats medicines as proprietary science, locking vaccines and drugs under market monopolies while numerous black and brown patients die.

We are witnessing a new form of medical apartheid in which preventable and curable diseases, such as TB, are thriving while lifesaving medicines remain in a stranglehold.

Unlike other diseases, the comeback of drug-resistant tuberculosis challenges the foundation of a story we have taken for granted: one of medicine's incremental advance and eventual triumph over pathogens.

The gains made in the twentieth century by medical science are being reversed in the twenty-first, during which the most powerful antibiotics known to humanity no longer work on this ancient and formidable foe.

The accompanying rise in authoritarianism, xenophobia, and science denialism combined with the regulatory capture of health resources by multinational corporations has created toxic and unique political circumstances that further enable viral and bacterial pathogens to thrive.

This book has one intended audience: readers who have the good fortune to have remained ignorant of TB but can ill afford to be so any longer.

PART I

CHAPTER 1

———◆———

THE GRAVE OF
MERCY BROWN

On a cold March morning in 1892, desperate to save his only surviving child, George Brown excavated the grave of his daughter. Mercy had died just two months earlier, at only nineteen years of age. She had been buried in the cemetery behind the Chestnut Hill Baptist Church in Exeter, Rhode Island.

Tumultuous events in Brown's life had led him to the ghastly task.

The previous fall, several members of his family had taken ill. Their symptoms—severe weight loss, night sweats, coughing up blood—were identical. Nothing he did helped them recover. Relatives and neighbors who remained healthy feared it was just a matter of time before they fell sick. The Exeter community had a meeting and voted on what to do next.

Increasingly terrified by the mysterious illness, the villagers turned to a mythical remedy popular at the time: if the heart of a corpse contained blood, it was believed that it was surviving off the blood and tissue of living family members—that the corpse was preying on the living. Since the afflicted showed similar symptoms, the villagers took that as proof that the dead were crawling out of their graves and consuming others, vampire style.

Most people in Exeter were convinced that three dead members of George Brown's family—his wife and two of their daughters, including Mercy—were draining the life of the last surviving child, Edwin, who had begun to show the all-too-familiar signs of approaching death.

When Edwin first fell ill, George had sent him to find a cure in the mineral waters of Colorado Springs, nearly two thousand miles west of the damp air of their home in coastal New England. It soon became clear that Edwin wasn't getting any better, and he was brought back home. Edwin's doctors could not explain his condition in the same way they had been unable to explain why his mother and sisters had died. They were clueless. When Edwin started to lose strength, color, and appetite, George Brown panicked.

Urged by friends and neighbors—who were convinced the deaths were caused by supernatural powers—George Brown turned to magical thinking and agreed to disinter and examine the bodies in the hope that the findings would calm the neighbors and George himself.

They were expecting to find that the bodies had naturally decomposed.

The town doctor, who attended the grisly exhumation, is said to have been the lone voice of reason that cold morning when the townspeople gathered in the Chestnut Hill cemetery.

Two days later, the exhumation of the dead Brown family was front-page news in the *Providence Journal*, Rhode Island's most widely read newspaper. It reported that Mrs. Brown and Mary Olive had mummified in the nine years they had spent in their graves.[1] Mrs. Brown's skeleton had some dried flesh and tissue remaining. Mary Olive's skull had a thick head of hair, but there was no sign of blood. The men then exhumed Mercy, who had died only two months earlier—on January 17, 1892. Mercy's body was fairly well preserved.

As was customary, her body had been kept aboveground in a crypt until the frozen earth had thawed enough to allow the digging of a proper grave. The doctor removed the heart and liver. The liver was dry, but the heart contained signs of decomposed, clotted blood. This was normal, considering the rate of decomposition during a frigid winter.

The *Providence Journal* filed another report on March 21, 1892:

> Dr. Harold Metcalf, the medical examiner of the district, who examined the bodies, is not one to believe in the vampire superstition. He made his examination, without exceptional results, according to his own belief, but found in one of the bodies, to the satisfaction of many of the people down there, a sign which they regarded as proof. When he removed the heart and liver from [Mercy's] body, a quantity of blood dripped therefrom, conforming to the theory of the necessity of destroying the vampire, burned the heart and liver.[2]

Edwin was given a potion mixed with some of the ashes of the burned offal as a possible antidote. Of course, it did not work.

He died four months later. This macabre episode gave birth to the legend of Mercy Brown, which in the annals of medical history is known as "The New England Vampire Panic."

In literary history, it is considered the origin of vampire fantasies, and Mercy became the inspiration for the most celebrated vampire victim of all, Lucy Westenra, in Bram Stoker's iconic Gothic horror novel, *Dracula*.

* * *

Before modern medicine, life was unpredictable, brutal, and, by extension, often short. Plagues were common, and the causes behind diseases such as yellow fever, smallpox, and malaria were unknown. What we do not understand, we fear.

In Exeter, people could *see* that the sickness in the Brown family was contagious. Three deaths in one family could not be a coincidence. They knew that whatever *it* was, it spread slowly but relentlessly. In this context, it is not difficult to understand why families would go to extreme lengths to find a "cure."

The exhumation of Mercy Brown did not occur in a vacuum.

With the advantage of hindsight and science, we now understand vampire panics as moments in human history when the inexorable power of superstition collided with emerging medical science.

Five years after Mercy Brown's exhumation, when Bram Stoker published *Dracula*, the book was more than a horror story. It referenced cutting-edge medical and scientific ideas of the time and wove in emerging technology of the late nineteenth century, such as photography, telephones, stenographs, and railroads.

Bram Stoker was fascinated by science, especially medical science. His uncle, William Stoker, was an eminent physician at the Cork Street Fever Hospital in Dublin, one of the most influential organizations studying infectious disease in the Victorian era. Stoker's older brother, Thornley, was a notable surgeon whose lectures on brain surgery appear in the notes for *Dracula*.[3] Stoker, in *Dracula*, captured the anxieties people felt about infectious diseases, including blood infections. Dracula himself is a centuries-old vampire and Transylvanian nobleman who is trying to move from Transylvania to England to find new blood and spread the curse of the undead. In London he discovers Lucy Westenra, who is perhaps not coincidentally the same age as Mercy Brown was when she died. Lucy is from a wealthy family, and Stoker's male-gaze-driven description of Lucy is "beautiful" and "angelic" but "simple-minded," with a singular ambition of finding a suitor.

She becomes Dracula's first victim, and he gradually drains the life from her with his vampiric attentions. Over the next month, doctors Abraham Van Helsing and John Seward try everything from blood transfusions to garlic blossoms, but Lucy keeps having "frightful relapses" until she dies.

At the funeral, Van Helsing notices that her canine teeth are longer than he remembered.

Soon after Lucy's death, there are reports of local children being attacked, all with the same "tiny wound" in the throat. On a hunch, Van Helsing goes to Lucy's grave only to find the coffin empty. She has risen from the grave, undead, and is feeding on a child. The men note that Lucy's sweetness has turned to "adamantine, heartless cruelty" and her purity to "voluptuous wantonness." To make sure Dracula does not revive her again, her head is chopped off and her mouth stuffed with garlic.

Only then is Lucy finally and permanently dead.

* * *

It is no coincidence that vampires, like pandemics, seem to come from elsewhere. Dracula was terrifying to urban London because he came from a remote, mountainous region of Eastern Europe, alien to most citizens of England's capital metropolis.

It is also not by chance that Dracula arrives in late August or September; that was also the season when cholera or bubonic plague had historically struck in Europe.

Like all aliens, Dracula faced a strong anti-immigrant sentiment.

The count is associated with swarms of rats and other creatures carrying filth and disease. The vampire brings a terrifying illness that thins the blood and corrupts the race. The book decries him as emerging from a "whirlpool" of races, a term Stoker borrows from late-Victorian debates, when it was used to describe the East End of London, home to large numbers of newly arrived Eastern European Jewish migrants who had fled from the pogroms. Their burgeoning numbers, swelling mainly in the slums, were feared to bring physical and moral infections to Britain.[4]

Vampires had been a part of ancient folklore long before Stoker's novel. English writer John William Polidori's 1819 short story "The Vampyre" is often credited with kick-starting the genre, something Stoker may have read as a teenager when he spent hours trawling through ancient, often illustrated texts of Irish folklore in Dublin's Marsh Library. But in *Dracula*, he gave the phenomenon a twist worthy of the Industrial Age.[5] *Dracula* is the Romanian word for "son of Dracul," a word that typically means "dragon" but can also mean "devil." Stoker's devil lived in Transylvania and traveled to London via ship and then railroad to reach London before he began ravaging the city. Both the vampire hunters in the novel—John Seward and Abraham Van Helsing—are doctors as well as experts in vampire lore, and they are on a mission to destroy the invader.

During this time, medical and literary opinion were often reflections of each other. *Dracula* is, essentially, a collection of

Victorian-era medical anxieties. It was written at a time when outbreaks ravaging British colonial outposts ended up at the doorsteps of the colonizers.

The most devastating example was the cholera pandemic of 1817, which began in faraway Bengal, India.

From India, cholera went to Southeast Asia, the Middle East, and eastern Africa through trade routes.[6] This was the first of several cholera pandemics to sweep through Asia and Europe during the nineteenth and twentieth centuries. The plague that began near Calcutta traveled the world for twenty years, killing hundreds of thousands. The exact death toll is unknown, but some data is preserved and suggests how vast the total number of deaths could have been. The British Army alone recorded ten thousand deaths, and the Indonesian island of Java recorded one million people dead.[7] To readers in London, the devil came from the east, as was customary.

Through the period of cholera outbreaks, there was ongoing debate in England about how diseases spread, and *Dracula* captured It perfectly when Stoker used blood infections as an integral element of his plot. In the Victorian era, many diseases that we now understand to be contagious (such as cholera and tuberculosis) were considered noncontagious.

In his forward-looking novel, Stoker went against mainstream medical views by building the myth of vampirism on the still-new concept of "infectious diseases": Dracula transmits the infection with a bite, leaving two puncture wounds, as if a snake had latched on to the neck. His victims are given blood transfusions, another pioneering technique that at the time was regarded as dangerous and experimental—which perhaps explains why Stoker's description of them is vague.

In the book, Seward states that Van Helsing performed the operation "with swiftness, but with absolute method." Beyond that, the actual task is left to the reader's imagination. Van Helsing describes Dracula's limitations and says, "It is said, too, that he can only pass running water at the slack or flood of the tide."[8] Since disease breeds in stagnant water, it makes sense that Dracula, the personification of disease, saw running water as a hostile environment.

Vampirism was an embodiment of disease.

One detail in the novel is most suggestive of the extent to which Bram Stoker was following contemporary medical thinking: the idea that a vampire can only rest in soil from the land of its origin.

Vampires need their native earth to survive. Dracula can only rest in a coffin filled with his native Transylvanian soil, which he has shipped from Eastern Europe for that purpose. To thwart him, one simply needs to destroy these boxes, which is what the doctors do in the novel. The doctors research extensively to understand their enemy, eventually isolate him, and eliminate the threat.

Van Helsing and the others locate forty-nine of the fifty boxes of soil transported to England and fill them with Eucharist wafers, supposedly purifying the soil and forcing Dracula to flee to his homeland.

Does it ring a bell?

Van Helsing and Seward are figuratively *sterilizing* Dracula's boxes of earth. They isolate the source of the "disease" to prevent transmission. It is good medical practice—but not yet common at the time.

Dracula's highly sexualized vampires and their fifty shades of red (especially his brides, who freely act on their sexual desires in exact opposition to men and women of the Victorian era) are often credited for capturing the repressed sexuality of the age. Films of the book emphasized these colorful aspects. But the novel did much more: *Dracula*, more than a century after it was published, remains relevant and provides a rare view of the enduring terror that mysterious infectious diseases had in the era before science.

* * *

Bram Stoker gained an intimate understanding of how devastating and mystifying infectious diseases can be from his mother, Charlotte Thornley Stoker.[9] She was born in 1818 and grew up in a pious Protestant family in Sligo, Ireland. She lived a life marked by tragedy, as she was born in the wake of a famine, which repeated with greater severity as she grew old.

It was not famine, however, that would leave an intergenerational scar on the Stoker family.

When Charlotte was fourteen years old, in 1832, she experienced a devastating cholera epidemic that killed more than half the population of the town. Bram grew up on her stories of the living being mistakenly buried with the dead in mass graves as cholera remorselessly claimed lives. She is known to have been one of Bram's trusted writing critics.

The cholera epidemic began in Calcutta in 1817, reaching Sligo by the summer of 1832. Sligo's residents watched tensely as the disease struck Dublin, Belfast, Limerick, and then the smaller towns: Tuam, Ballinrobe, and Castlebar. Just when the people of Sligo thought they had been spared, the first victim died on August 11—the same date that Dracula claims Lucy, his first victim in London.

In just six weeks, an estimated fifteen hundred townspeople died from the disease. Deaths were estimated at around an astonishing fifty per day, and some estimate the total death toll to be around eighteen hundred during the epidemic, which lasted from August to September.

Charlotte's family escaped, but she was forever haunted by what she witnessed.

In 1873, she would finally narrate her trauma in a paper titled "Experiences of the Cholera in Ireland." It is likely that Bram persuaded her to finally put on paper the stories she had told him throughout his childhood. In eleven pages, Charlotte provides a blueprint for Dracula.

Many of her observations found their way into her son's novel. She noted that people in Sligo believed that cholera affected port towns and that it traveled by ship. When the epidemic eventually ended, she recalled that there remained a terrible smell in the town for months after.

In *Dracula*, places associated with the count have a rotting smell. Charlotte said it was believed cholera traveled as a mist over land; Count Dracula too can change into a mist. Charlotte noted that people spoke of weird weather conditions—unusual storms, thunder, and lightning—in Sligo before cholera made its appearance, and the same atmospherics dominate the book. As Sligo's fever hospital was overwhelmed, residents noticed that the Catholic clergy were not reporting as many casualties, despite being in contact with the afflicted. They were thought to be, miraculously, immune to cholera. In *Dracula*, this would show up as symbols of Roman Catholicism, such as holy water and the crucifix, becoming useful tools to fight vampirism.

The most significant influence, however, would come from the grim details about live burials. Charlotte wrote about the victims being buried within hours of death in mass graves for fear of the spread of the disease.

In haste, many people were buried before they had died.

Early in the epidemic in Sligo, Charlotte recounts the story of a victim who "awoke" while the undertaker was trying to fit him into the coffin. A second man pulled his wife's body from a mass grave for a proper burial, only to discover she was still alive. "He sought her body to give it a more decent burial than could be given there, (the custom was to dig a large trench, put forty or fifty without coffins, throw lime on them and cover the grave). He saw the corner of his red handkerchief under several bodies, which he removed, found his wife and found that there was still life. He carried her home, and she recovered and lived many years."[10] While Stoker never divulged his inspirations, in a rare 1897 interview, he admitted that *Dracula* was inspired by the idea of "someone being buried before they were fully dead." His working title of the book had actually been *The Undead*; the publisher changed it to *Dracula* prior to publication.

* * *

Mercy Brown's exhumation became the most publicized of a long series of "vampire panics." New England was not the only place to have experienced a rash of vampire burials. The American phenomenon went on for nearly a hundred years, starting in the late 1700s, and was preceded by European outbreaks.

In March 2009, the corpse of an elderly woman dubbed the Vampire of Venice was found buried in a sixteenth-century plague pit, with a brick jammed between her jaws.[11] Italian researchers believe she had been buried so brutally to prevent her from feeding on the victims of a plague that was sweeping the city. Gravediggers would sometimes come across bodies bloated by gas, with hair still growing and blood seeping from their mouths, and believe them to be still alive or undead.

Shrouds used to cover the faces of the dead were often decayed by bacteria in the mouth, revealing the corpse's teeth; thus, vampires became known as "shroud-eaters." According to medieval medical and religious texts, the undead were believed to spread pestilence in order to suck the remaining life from corpses until they acquired the strength to return to the streets. The general wisdom was that to kill the vampire, you had to remove the shroud from its mouth, which was its food, and replace it with something inedible, like a brick.

In the 1850s, decades before Mercy Brown was dug up, there was a similar panic in Jewitt City, Connecticut.

This time, the Ray family was at the eye of the storm.

Formerly robust family members were carried to the grave, and just like the Browns, the Rays helplessly watched their loved ones waste away.

The stories of the two families are nearly interchangeable.

Over the course of nine years, the Rays lost multiple family members to the same symptoms. The first to die was twenty-four-year-old Lemuel in 1845; less than four years later, patriarch Henry was felled. He was followed to the grave by twenty-six-year-old Elisha in 1851. Three short years later, in 1854, the eldest son, also named Henry, was struck by the now all-too-familiar symptoms, and this was when the panic truly set in. Just like George Brown, the Rays realized their neighbors' talk in the village had become not altogether friendly. The family decided something drastic had to be done, and quickly.

Two of the sons—Lemuel and Elisha—were exhumed on June 8, 1854.[12] According to newspaper accounts, the decomposing bodies were dug up and burned immediately. It is unclear why their father's grave was spared, but by all indications, the exhumation had done the trick. The son named Henry survived his affliction, unlike Edwin Brown. The family believed exhuming and burning the bodies had stopped the vampire, and the method caught on.

In neighboring Hopeville, the Walton family was going through a similar crisis. They lived less than two miles from the Rays' farm and had heard of how the Rays had stopped the deaths: by destroying the dead to spare the living.

For 136 years, no one would know of the Walton family's struggles until, in November 1990, children playing on an eroding hillside discovered an unmarked grave.

A police investigation was launched, as they initially believed the grave has been dug by a serial killer. Forensic archaeologists conducted a yearlong excavation and eventually found a total of twenty-nine unmarked graves.

One of the graves, named Burial #4, stood out.

The entombment contained a coffin with "JB-55" spelled in brass tacks on the lid and was different from all the others. The skeleton they found was not white but painted red. The bones belonged to a male between fifty and fifty-five years old who had died in the early to mid-1800s. The feet were exactly where you'd expect them to be, but the rest of the body had been rearranged. The skull was in a "Jolly Roger" arrangement, with face turned downward and a pair of femur bones placed just below in an X.

The researchers found that JB-55 had been dismembered about five years after death, with the positioning of the bones suggesting there was very little soft tissue left on the corpse when it was unearthed. That meant there were no organs to burn to stop vampiric activity. The archaeologists maintain that the corpse was beheaded as an alternative to burning the heart.[13] Forensics revealed the cause of death as consumption.

Two other graves, named IB-45 and NB-13 (the numbers are indicators of the age), contained the remains of people who had died of the same illness.

Consumption, a historical name for the mysterious illness, is an apt description of the symptoms. The afflicted started coughing up blood; grew feverish and pale; and rapidly lost strength, appetite, and weight, leaving an impression that life is being slowly sucked away, or consumed.

Through the 1800s, the diagnosis of consumption was a death sentence.

In 1892, the year Mercy died, the American civil war had greatly reduced Exeter's population, and railroads had made it possible for residents to migrate to the countryside in search of better farmland and economic opportunity. Between 1820 and 1892, Exeter's population fell from 2,500 to 961.[14] Families were barely getting by when they also started dropping dead from the strange illness. The twelve biggest vampire-related exhumations in eighteenth- and nineteenth-century New England—in Connecticut, Vermont, Rhode Island, and Massachusetts—all turned out to be of people whose deaths resulted from consumption. The epidemic, also described as the "Great White Plague"—after the anemic pallor of patients as they wasted away—actually began eating away at humans over nine thousand years ago. Though the panics eventually stopped, consumption did not.

The Great White Plague has left an indelible mark on human civilization, with traces found in Egyptian mummies dating back to 2400 BC. Medical historians speculate that consumption began in the first cities of the ancient world and that the ancient Egyptians may have bequeathed on the world—in addition to civilization—this malignancy.

The ancient Greeks called it phthisis (pronounced "thay-sis"), meaning "wasting away." In ancient Rome it was called scrofula, and in India it was referred to as *yaksma*, with the first reference in non-European civilization found in *Rigveda* (around 1500 BC).

This disease, among the oldest in the world, has been a parallel to history itself.

Consumption is a remarkably enduring disease. Once it arrives, it stays. It ravages cities and plunders populations, and for that it was called the "Captain of All These Men of Death" by English writer John Bunyan in his 1680 novel, *The Life and Death of Mr. Badman*.

Today, we know the disease as tuberculosis.

Vampire panics can be explained away as the reaction of the uneducated, frightened masses from an era before modern medical science. Our rituals are not the same in the twenty-first century; nevertheless, when confronted by an incurable disease, we continue to react with manic alarm and often with the same hysteria George Brown showed that March morning in Exeter, standing over the grave of his daughter.

CHAPTER 2

DR. IGNAZ SEMMELWEIS, SAVIOR OF MOTHERS

The knowledge that boiling water kills germs and handwashing prevents disease was not accepted in nineteenth-century Europe, when doctors arrived at the operating table in their street clothes and, without washing their hands or putting on scrubs or surgical gloves, set to work on their often unlucky patients.

Sterilization was also unknown; if a scalpel fell to the ground during an operation, it would be picked up and reused. In the world before the invention of microscopes, the idea of germs was as invisible as the germs themselves.

One of the most common causes of death among women at that time was a devastating infection called puerperal or "childbed" fever, a postpartum infection in the uterus. The infection is now largely preventable due to infection-control practices and, when it does occur, is easily treated, thanks to antibiotics. Until recently, pregnant women dreaded labor; childbed fever was a near certainty.

Within three days of giving birth, patients often developed abdominal pain, fever, and infection, quickly resulting in death. It affected everyone—the wives of prime ministers and kings were as susceptible as other women. Jane Seymour, queen of England from 1536 to 1537, and the third wife of King Henry VIII, died of it, nine days after delivering Princess Elizabeth.[1] Childbed fever became deadlier in the nineteenth century due to two changes: more babies were delivered in the hospital instead of at home, making it easier for the infection to spread around the wards, and autopsies began to be conducted on childbed-fever victims to understand the cause of the disease. With the lack of sterilization practices, the doctor conducting the autopsy often became infected and went on, unwittingly, to transmit the infection to other patients.

Eventually a luckless doctor, ahead of his time, discovered the cause. His ideas saved millions of lives, sparing countless mothers and newborns from excruciating deaths. For that, he was initially demoted, eventually fired, and committed to a mental asylum, where he died after being beaten to death while trying to escape.

In the nineteenth century, when maternal and infant mortality rates averaged 50 percent, the immovable ideas of formal medicine collided with newly discovered scientific evidence.

The man at the center of it all was Ignaz Semmelweis.[2]

* * *

Our tragic hero was born in 1818 to Teresia Müller and Josef Semmelweis on July 1. The family of German Jewish immigrants to Hungary ran a grocery shop successful enough to allow them to afford an education for all eight of their children.[3] Ignaz, the fifth child, grew up in a reasonably happy home in the district of old Buda called Tabán. The city, in 1873, combined with Pest and Óbuda to form Budapest. At this time, Buda was administered as part of the Austrian Empire.

The building where the Semmelweis family lived still stands on Aprod Street as a museum for the history of medicine and holds several objects belonging to the Semmelweises. Among them is a diary of a friend of the family, which states that young Ignaz was "happy, truthful, open-minded and extremely popular with friends and colleagues."[4] By all accounts, he was an incredibly intelligent child and "one of the most cheerful, life-affirming and carefree students in Vienna." He threw himself into his education with "immeasurable ambition and extraordinary diligence, perseverance and exactitude."[5]

Ignaz came to obstetrics in a roundabout way. He began studying law at the University of Vienna in the autumn of 1837. By the following year, for unknown reasons, he switched to medicine. He was awarded a master's degree in midwifery in 1844 and became a surgeon in 1845.

After failing to obtain an appointment in a clinic for internal medicine, Semmelweis decided to specialize in obstetrics, then considered a lowly branch of medicine.

A year later he joined the maternity clinic of the Vienna General Hospital, a teaching hospital and one of the busiest institutions in the world at the time. It was not a prestigious posting, nor was it his first choice, but the newly qualified Dr. Semmelweis threw himself into the routine of a busy physician.

On his twenty-eighth birthday, in 1846, Dr. Semmelweis was granted a two-year appointment as assistant to physician Johannes Klein, director of the Vienna General Hospital; thus began the obsession that would consume his life.

Working in the maternity clinic of a teaching hospital meant that Semmelweis had to perform two roles: teacher and doctor.

He inspected patients in the morning and prepared them for the bedside rounds undertaken by the senior doctors and assisted the doctors during obstetric surgeries. He also taught medical students obstetrics by demonstrating procedures on corpses, and he was in charge of statistical records as the "cleric of record," which put him in the perfect position to spot death patterns among patients.

The Viennese Maternity Clinic was set up specifically to serve the poor, including prostitutes. At that time, desperately poor mothers often used infanticide—the intentional killing of babies—as a method of "birth control."[6] To stop this, the government offered free care to pregnant women, setting up institutions like the Viennese clinic. The clinics would look after the infants, and in return the women would be subjects for the training of doctors and midwives.

In 1841, due to growing numbers of patients, the hospital opened a second obstetrics clinic for the instruction of midwives alone. Most doctors in that period were men. Women, as nurses and midwives, were not allowed into the universities and could not gain a license to practice medicine.

At Dr. Semmelweis's clinic, male students who were being trained to become doctors practiced their medicine on patients, having tried out their skills on autopsies; midwives, educated in the second clinic, did not conduct autopsies.

That would make all the difference.

Almost as soon as the clinics were segregated, the difference in deaths from childbed fever between the two increased dramatically. Semmelweis noticed this immediately as the cleric of record.[7] He was shocked to learn that the mortality rate of those treated in the first clinic, run by doctors, was at one point as high as 10 percent. The second clinic, run by midwives, had an average mortality rate of less than 4 percent.[8] News of the disparity soon spread.

The two clinics admitted patients on alternate days. Semmelweis described women begging on their knees not to be admitted to the first clinic and that some women even preferred to give birth in the streets, *pretending* to have gone into labor while en route to the hospital.[9] It meant they would still qualify for the child-care benefits without being admitted. To Semmelweis's horror, the women delivering in the streets had a better survival rate than the women admitted to the first clinic. Most of his colleagues chalked up the deaths in the first clinic to bad air, or foul smells, which drove Semmelweis to despair: "It made me so miserable," he wrote, "that life seemed worthless."[10]

Semmelweis concluded that whatever was going wrong in the first clinic was because of something inside it. Doctors there were using the same techniques but causing more deaths, and he was determined to find out why. He first meticulously eliminated *all* possible differences; for example, the same laundry contractor would henceforth wash the linen from both clinics, and the same food would be served to all patients.

In his obsession to keep patients alive, he picked a fight with everyone else—just the kind of doctor every patient wants. He was extremely strict and was once noted to have used "mild corporal punishment" to discipline a laundry owner who brought back the patients' sheets stained with blood and pus.[11]

He was kind to his patients though.

As part of his investigations, he also looked into the religious practices of those working in the clinics. According to accepted Catholic rituals of the time, a priest would be summoned from the hospital chapel to administer last rites. Every time the priest came, a sacristan—a person in charge of sacristy—would ring a bell. For expecting mothers in the two clinics, this bell was an audible reminder of the horrors that lay ahead.

Thinking the bell might trigger the patients emotionally (pan-icked patients do worse medically), Semmelweis asked that the use of bells be stopped. Eventually, both clinics were run and operated identically in every respect; however, the death rates in the first clinic remained high.

Meanwhile, Semmelweis's authoritarian manner saw him demoted.

Up until this point in history, it was maintained that disease spread because of bad air, characterized by its foul smell. This was known as the "miasmatic theory," originating in the Middle Ages. *Miasma* is the ancient Greek term for pollution. The miasmatic theory, which also gave rise to the naming of malaria (literally meaning "bad air" in medieval Italian), held that diseases such as cholera, infections such as chlamydia, or plagues such as the Black Death were caused by a *miasma*.

Dracula, for that reason, was surrounded by miasma. The mist surrounding the count, and the garlic flowers that repel him, are suggestions of miasmatic belief. In Stoker's *Dracula*, when Jonathan Harker visits the count's room in Transylvania, he smells "a deathly, sickly odour."[12] The book consistently refers to this sense of decay suspended in the air in the presence of the vampire.

Stoker used miasmatic imagery to convey the horror of illness.

Until the mid-nineteenth century, the medical community believed epidemics were caused by something nasty in the air, and the theory was extended to other conditions. It was believed that you could become obese by inhaling the odor of food. The other popular explanation for disease was called "spontaneous generation," a little like the immaculate conception. The Greek philosopher Aristotle (384–322 BC) was one of the earliest recorded scholars to articulate the notion that life can arise from nonliving matter. It held that different types of life might repeatedly emerge from specific sources other than seeds or eggs.

Yet as early as the sixteenth century, an Italian scholar and physician named Girolamo Fracastoro had floated the idea of contagion—that small, invisible organisms were causing diseases.[13]

Like most new ideas, his views were held in disdain.

A century later another Italian physician, Francesco Redi, provided evidence against "spontaneous generation," a belief that flies spontaneously generated from rotting meat.[14] In 1668, he devised an experiment in which he placed meat in three jars. One of the jars was left open, another one tightly sealed, and the last one covered with gauze.

After a few days, he observed that the meat in the open jar was covered by maggots, and the jar covered with gauze had maggots on the outside surface of the gauze. The tightly sealed jar had no maggots inside or outside it. He also noticed that the maggots were found only on surfaces that were accessible to flies.

A few years later, in 1676, Dutchman Antonie van Leeuwenhoek observed bacteria and other microorganisms in water, the first to be observed by man, using a single-lens microscope of his own design.[15] Leeuwenhoek, commonly known as "the father of microscopy," is central to the story of one of the most significant developments in the history of science.

The nature of scientific discovery has always been one of incremental advances, based on achievements of men like van Leeuwenhoek, Redi, and Semmelweis. Examples of this abound in the histories of science and medicine. We prefer the single story of a genius with a game-changing eureka moment, but in truth the revolutionary scientific progress made by flamboyant doctors like Louis Pasteur, Joseph Lister, and Robert Koch was possible only because they were standing on the shoulders of men like Redi, van Leeuwenhoek, and Semmelweis.

Semmelweis, despite his demotion, was still intent on discovering the reasons for the mortality-rate discrepancies between the first and second clinics and dismissed his colleagues' explanations of miasma being the cause. They said deaths in the first clinic were due to overcrowding and the resultant foul smell; however, the clerical records showed that the second clinic was, in fact, the one that was overcrowded, with the women who were trying to avoid being admitted to the first clinic, where they knew they were more likely to die.

Tortured by the mystery, Semmelweis took a trip to Venice along with two of his friends, hoping that "the Venetian art treasures would revive my mind and spirits, which have been so seriously affected by my experiences in the maternity hospital."[16] When he returned to Vienna, he was shocked to find that a dear friend and colleague, Jakob Kolletschka, had died after accidentally being poked with a student's scalpel while performing a postmortem examination on a patient who had died of childbed fever. Kolletschka's own autopsy revealed a cause of death similar to those of childbed fever victims.

Semmelweis immediately made a far-reaching connection and set about conducting a series of experiments. After a year, he finally understood the crucial difference between the two clinics: the midwives, unlike doctors who performed autopsies, had no contact with cadavers. Typically, the doctors would perform autopsies in the morning, barehanded; then, without washing their hands, they would head into the maternity ward to deliver babies. Semmelweis concluded that doctors carried "cadaverous particles" from the autopsy room to the patients they examined. When they delivered the babies, these particles would get inside the women.

If his hypothesis proved to be correct, getting rid of the cadaverous particles would reduce the death rate from childbed fever.

By the end of May 1847, two months after his return from Venice, Semmelweis instituted a policy of using a chlorinated solution for handwashing and the cleaning of instruments before the examination of patients and after autopsy work.

In a repeat of the move that led to his demotion, Semmelweis ruled that all first-clinic physicians must also wash their hands with chlorinated lime. His colleagues chafed at the idea, literally, as bleach is irritating to the skin.

Semmelweis didn't know anything about germs. He chose chlorine because he thought it would be the best way to get rid of any smells left behind by those little bits of corpse. It was good fortune that he chose one of the best disinfectants, but it was to clear the air.

With the new handwashing routine in place, the death rate in the first clinic began to drop. It had been 18 percent in April and went down to 2 percent by June. In August, for the first time ever, no one died of childbed fever in the doctors' clinic.

Semmelweis had solved the problem without being able to explain why handwashing and sterilizing made the difference. Nonetheless, he stubbornly insisted that other physicians unquestioningly follow his rules until he could find the answer. His colleagues, who did not like him to begin with, took this as a personal attack. They grumbled about how unthinkable it was to accuse prestigious physicians of being carriers of contagion, a theory for which Semmelweis could offer no evidence.

It did not help that Semmelweis enforced his new rules and monitored their hygiene with characteristic authoritarian impulse. He assigned a midwife and a medical student to each patient. The student's name was publicly displayed so Semmelweis could immediately identify if anyone skipped handwashing. He also demanded that the students wash and sterilize their medical instruments.

Despite the unpopularity of his new rules, the statistics were clear, and by the end of the year, talk of his experiments was spreading across Europe. Semmelweis, who had only been in the position of senior resident at the clinic for eighteen months, had every hope that his practices would be globally accepted.

However, he did not publish a paper about his findings. Never the crowd pleaser, he disliked public speaking and writing, which made it difficult to secure recognition for his discovery and went against the grain of academia's long-standing "publish or perish" culture. With the concept of germs yet to be discovered, Semmelweis lacked the framework to explain his breakthrough. The lack of explanation became a reason to argue against his discovery.

Semmelweis soon became adamant, to a degree that inevitably caused offence. He started publicly berating people who disagreed with him, and he made influential enemies. Eventually the doctors gave up the chlorine handwashing, and Semmelweis lost his job.

Making matters worse, the year after his breakthrough, in 1848, there was an uprising in Vienna against the Austrian Empire, and Hungarians, like the Semmelweis family, began to be mistrusted. Although there is no evidence that Semmelweis was a part of the revolution, many of his students and at least one of his siblings were.

In 1850, he left the city without saying goodbye to anyone. He returned to Hungary and for the next decade faced relentless ridicule for his ideas about handwashing. Semmelweis, now without a job and infuriated, started writing open letters to prominent obstetricians, accusing them of being murderers.

In 1861, he wrote about it: "Most medical lecture halls continue to resound with lectures on epidemic childbed fever and with discourses against my theories. . . . In published medical works my teachings are either ignored or attacked. The medical faculty at Würzburg awarded a prize to a monograph written in 1859 in which my teachings were rejected."[17] Semmelweis's research and style were too radical and too impolite. His ideas, like him, were an affront to the self-esteem of illustrious doctors of the gentleman classes. His method of using statistics as medical evidence was not then understood or accepted. The centuries-old thesis that this disease was spread by miasma or contagium was too deeply rooted.

Semmelweis, isolated and mocked, was not, however, entirely alone. At some point in the same decade, thankfully for all humanity, French, German, and English scientists walked into their labs.

* * *

The story of germ theory, like all good stories, is one of incrementality.

As Semmelweis was struggling to explain the idea of contagion, a younger scientist in France was toying with a similar problem—but from a completely different angle. In 1845—the same year Semmelweis became a surgeon—Louis Pasteur, twenty-three years old, graduated with a degree of licencié ès sciences (MS) from the École Normale Supérieure.[18] He would spend the next two decades studying chemistry and fermentation.

In May 1849, Pasteur married Marie Laurent, the daughter of the rector of the university. The couple had five children; only two survived childhood. In 1859, when they lost a daughter to typhoid, Pasteur threw himself into his work, turning his attention to "wine maladies."

French wine was prized around Europe, and a trade deal with Britain dramatically boosted French wine exports; however, much of it spoiled during transit, souring instead of fermenting. The "wine maladies" became a national crisis, and eager to save the country's reputation and economy, emperor Napoleon III asked Pasteur, by now a famous chemist, to figure out what was happening and fix the problem.

Pasteur realized that boiling wine to kill bacteria made it taste terrible. After a series of experiments, he discovered that by heating wine precisely to 131 degrees Fahrenheit, he could kill the bacteria but not ruin the taste. Pasteur had, early on, sided with the minority point of view among his contemporaries: that fermentation was caused by a living microorganism and not spontaneously generated. His study of wine contamination helped prove the point, showing it to be caused by microbes.

This thunderbolt of an idea—the beginning of "germ theory"— saved the wine industry from collapse, but its impact was much greater. Pasteur realized the fermentation process caused by bacteria was similar to the infections found in wounds. He was the first to imagine disease as a process that involved living things. Understanding the enormity of his discovery, he famously said, "A bottle of wine contains more philosophy than all the books in the world."

Germ theory was inherently controversial, but especially because the idea was coming from a chemist, not a doctor. The genius of Pasteur was that he made two far-reaching connections: that the fermentation in wine (or infection) was caused by living things and that this could be controlled by heat. What we now know as the process of pasteurization is a result of this discovery and has saved countless lives around the world.

The idea was a paradigm shift.

Germ theory was to medicine what Italian astronomer Galileo Galilei's theory on earth's rotation was to astronomy or Sir Isaac Newton's theory of gravitation was to physics or Charles Darwin's theory of natural selection was to biology. It changed every single concept, theory, and standard for what had constituted the legitimate practice of medicine. However, like all radical ideas, it was widely debated and repeatedly rejected until it became impossible to reject anymore.

The process would take three decades and cost countless lives.

After his discovery of the effect of heat on bacteria, Pasteur moved on to take down another beloved medical superstition, spontaneous generation, which had led to all sorts of magical thinking: that dust creates fleas, that maggots arise from rotting meat, and that bread or wheat left in a dark corner could produce mice.[19] In 1861, Pasteur gave a lecture, "On Organized Corpuscles That Exist in the Atmosphere; Examination of the Doctrine of Spontaneous Generation," that proved conclusively that infection was not spontaneously generated, that in fact infection and many diseases were caused by bacteria.

Once again, at the request of the French government, Pasteur conducted a series of experiments, this time turning his attention to silkworm disease, which was attacking the French silkworm nurseries. It would be his entry into the world of infectious diseases.[20]

In the middle of the nineteenth century, a mysterious disease had attacked French silkworm nurseries. Silkworm eggs could no longer be produced in France, and they could not be imported from other countries, as the same disease had spread to other silk-producing countries, such as Italy, Austria, and the Ottoman

Empire. By 1865, this crisis had become a matter of national economic interest.

By now, Pasteur was going through one of the roughest phases of his life. His second daughter died of typhus in 1865 at two years old; a third daughter, aged twelve, died from a tumor in 1866; and in 1868, at forty-five, Pasteur suffered a stroke that partially paralyzed his left side.[21] Still, he did not stop his research. His colleagues set up a mobile laboratory that allowed him to work from his sickbed. After five years, he succeeded in saving the silk industry by discovering a method that enabled the preservation of healthy silkworm eggs and prevented their contamination by disease-causing organisms. He established that healthy worms became ill when they nested in the bedding of diseased worms, that environment directly led to contagion, and that the spread of disease could be controlled by sterilization.

He convincingly linked contagion to a specific disease.

This led to a new phase of discoveries that made the closing decades of the nineteenth century a golden era of medical science. Pasteur's considerable renown caught the attention of an English scientist, Joseph Lister, a professor of surgery at Edinburgh University and an unlikely hero whose discoveries, when combined with those of Semmelweis and Pasteur, would change the world.

Lister was the second of three children born to Isabella Harris and Joseph Jackson Lister, a successful wine merchant and amateur scientist.[22] Young Lister was mild-mannered, courteous, and not keen on confrontation. He had soft blue eyes and a pleasant and gentle smile. He spoke softly, frequently with a slight stammer, and sighed often.[23] The world of surgery was still primitive.

In *The Butchering Art*, the historian Lindsey Fitzharris reveals the grisly world of nineteenth-century medicine. The surgeries were done without anesthesia and had to be done quickly, lest the patient bleed to death. Doctors took pride in their speed and brute strength, using the most primitive of tools that today would not look out of place in a garden shed.

Then there were postsurgery infections to contend with, made worse by the fact that doctors wore aprons that had so much dried blood on them, they could stand on their own. Bed linen and laboratory coats went unwashed, and surgical instruments were cleaned only before they were put away for storage. Surgeons of the time referred to the "good old surgical stink" and took pride in the stains on their unwashed operating gowns as a display of their experience.

Semmelweis's now-legendary work on childbed fever had by then fallen into obscurity.

While everyone around him considered it a status symbol to be covered in blood from previous operations, Lister washed his hands before operating and wore clean clothes.[24] He demonstrated a rare compassion for patients and urged that every patient be treated "with the same care and regard" as if they were the prince of Wales. When a young girl, whom Lister had treated for an abscess on her knee, presented the surgeon with her rag doll and its detached leg, he threaded a needle and sewed it back on.[25] Lister was appalled by the number of patients who died after otherwise successful surgeries. This period seems to be the origin of the tired medical joke: operation successful, patient dead.

Because of the high rate of mortality from hospital infections, surgeries were performed only as a last resort. There was talk of banning all surgery from hospitals because of septic complications. Sir J. E. Erichsen, a future president of the Royal College of Surgeons, stated, "The abdomen, chest, and brain will forever be closed to operations by a wise and humane surgeon."[26] A broken leg, while painful, is not something that often causes death today. Around 150 years ago, this was not the case. A broken leg meant amputation, and in about half of such cases, the patient subsequently died of infection.

Joseph Lister helped put an end to this tragic waste of life, the same way Semmelweis did with childbed fever.

Lister realized that broken bones healed without infection when the skin was not broken—whereas compound fractures (when bones pierce through the skin) often became infected. Lister reasoned that somehow the infection was entering the wound from the outside, that the infecting agent was something in the air.

Like Semmelweis, he did not know exactly how this happened.

As the son of a wine merchant, Lister was all too familiar with the problem of wine going sour due to fermentation. His great intellectual breakthrough came when, on the advice of Thomas Anderson, a professor of chemistry at Glasgow University, he read Pasteur's *Recherches sur la putréfaction* and postulated that the same process causing fermentation was involved with wound sepsis.[27] Lister was struck by Pasteur's ideas and reached the next logical conclusion: that airborne germs caused wound infections after operations. It was after reading of Louis Pasteur's discovery of microscopic objects—bacteria—in sour wine that the penny dropped.

Lister then took another logical leap of faith: that infections were not caused by the chemical reaction of oxidation, or in other words, wounds do not become septic just because they have been touched by air. They become infected (or contaminated) because of living microorganisms. Lister started washing his hands and sterilizing his instruments before operations.

After various experiments with cleansing chemicals, Lister opted for carbolic acid, used in sewage works to counter bad smells.

Then, in August 1865, after two failed efforts, Lister performed an operation to mend the broken leg of an eleven-year-old boy, James Greenlees, who had been hit by a cart. The boy had a compound fracture of the lower left leg. He was given chloroform, and Lister washed the wound out and applied a dressing of carbolic acid (now called phenol) as a disinfectant. A splint and bandages were put in place, and the carbolic acid dressing was renewed several times as the days went by. The wound began to scab over and heal. After six weeks Greenlees was discharged, fully recovered, and left Glasgow Royal Infirmary completely cured.[28] It was Lister's first success. It took another two years of research before Lister felt ready to share his findings, in a five-part report published in 1867 in the *Lancet*. From then on, Lister laid out the protocol for sterilizing surgical instruments, surgeons' hands, dressings, and wounds with solutions of carbolic acid and even designed a sprayer to diffuse the substance in the foul-smelling air of the operating room.

Yet despite his findings, and despite the findings of Semmelweis and Pasteur, the idea of invisible germs floating in the air was mocked by a majority of the medical community, who considered it unscientific quackery. The editor of the magazine *Medical Record* wrote, "We are likely to be as much ridiculed in the next century for our blind belief in the power of unseen germs, as our forefathers were for their faith in the influence of spirits, of certain planets and the like, inducing certain maladies."[29]

The story of the acceptance of germ theory would not be complete without another hero of science: Robert Koch.

Robert Heinrich Hermann Koch was born on December 11, 1843, in Clausthal, Germany. The son of a mining engineer, he demonstrated a gifted mind at an early age, reportedly announcing to his parents at the age of five that he had taught himself to read by using newspapers.[30] In 1862, Koch went to the University of Göttingen to study medicine. Here the professor of anatomy was Jacob Henle, and Koch was, no doubt, influenced by Henle's view, published in 1840, that infectious diseases were caused by living, parasitic organisms.

Despite the advances made by the heroes of this story, it would be another decade before Koch's idea inflicted a final, mortal blow to the notions of spontaneous generation and miasma theory. When Koch started practicing, the majority view in the medical community—driven by ego, largely—was to disregard scientific evidence and continue to believe in the theory of miasma.

Koch graduated from university in 1866; married his home-town sweetheart, Emma Fraatz, the following year; and saw the birth of his only child, Gertrud, fourteen months later.[31] His first microscope, a gift from his wife, was a source of great joy.[32] Four years later, on July 19, 1870, the Franco-Prussian War broke out, lasting until May 10, 1871. A coalition of German states led by Prussia outmanned and outmaneuvered France, marking the end of French hegemony in Europe. It also led to the creation of uni-fied Germany. The war involved around two million soldiers and resulted in the deaths of more than 180,000 men. Pasteur's son was among the wounded. Koch had volunteered for medical service in the war, which set the stage for an epic scientific feud—one that would go on to eventually benefit humanity.

This era in medical discovery was, in a way, similar to the Cold War–era space race. The germ theory was hotly debated, and every leading scientist wanted to get in on it. Like many of his fellow young physicians, Koch was struck by an intense fascination with all things microscopic, a fixation some medical critics derided as "bacteriomania." Pasteur, who was by now a celebrity scientist with a huge fan base, also knew how to ride on the wave of nationalism and cultivate the media.

Fans of Pasteur were rivaled by the fans of Koch, twenty years younger than Pasteur. The most famous Frenchman of his generation, Pasteur was a chemist with a broad philosophical interest in microbial science. Koch, by contrast, was a physician principally interested in microbial (especially bacterial) causes of human disease.

If Pasteur's genius was imagination, Koch's was rigor.

Although Koch's initial encounter with Pasteur in London was cordial, he soon began attacking his rival in writing. In particular, Koch accused Pasteur of using impure cultures and of conducting faulty inoculation studies. This infuriated the French public.

Pasteur responded by sending his assistant, Louis Thuillier, to Prussia to demonstrate his techniques. Thuillier wrote, "Koch is not liked by his colleagues. . . . [He] is a bit of a rustic, and is ignorant of parliamentary language."[33] Koch traded insults: "Pasteur is not a physician, and one cannot expect him to make sound judgments about pathological processes and the symptoms of disease."

The rivalry had both harmful and beneficial effects.

In France, it delayed acceptance of the culture techniques promoted by Koch; in Germany, Pasteur's newly discovered vaccine against rabies was slow to be put into use. Yet the competition between the two, animated by an intense desire to garner the highest accolades of scientific achievement, led to indisputable accomplishments that would outlive the feud. In 1875, Koch visited many of Germany's great scientific research centers, which attuned him to the emerging world of microbial science. Louis Pasteur had discovered that bacteria cause putrefaction; Joseph Lister had developed techniques of antiseptic surgery; and Jacob Henle, Koch's anatomy teacher in Göttingen, was defending the idea of *contagium animatum*, which held that disease could be caused by living transferable entities.

The future of miasmatic theory and spontaneous generation was finally precarious.

After returning from service in the Franco-Prussian War, Koch worked as a district medical officer. In 1880, he was appointed a member of the Imperial Health Bureau in Berlin and for the first time in his life had access to a superb laboratory, powerful microscopes, animals to be used for experiments, and assistants.

He decided to try to find the cause of one of the major killers of his day: tuberculosis—a controversial choice. Most experts insisted that TB was a hereditary disease; after all, it did tend to "run" in families.[34] He ignored them and became the first person to isolate the specific bacteria that caused TB. To simplify, if Pasteur said germs caused disease, it was Koch who said mycobacterium *tuberculosis* caused TB—he linked a specific germ to a specific disease. He also laid down four rules, known as Koch's postulates, which he argued must be satisfied before it could be accepted that a particular bacteria caused a particular disease:

1. The microorganism (or "pathogen") must be in all animals suffering from this disease. It has to be found where the disease is.
2. The microorganism must be able to be isolated and grown in culture.
3. The microorganism must cause the disease when introduced in a different, healthy animal.

4. The microorganism must be able to be reisolated from the infected animal and match with the organism from the first animal.

These postulates established *causality* for the first time and put germ theory on solid ground.

Pasteur's crowning achievement was to prove germs caused disease, but the practical question was, Which specific germs caused what disease, and how could they be stopped? Koch took that next logical step in the journey toward modern medicine.

On March 24, 1882, in a lecture hall at the Physiological Society of Berlin, Koch delivered one of the most famous medical lectures of all time. He announced that he had found a bacterium—*tubercle bacillus*—that caused TB.

Since the disease was decimating the population, this announcement was one of the most sensational events in medical history.

Koch was not a dynamic speaker, and on this day he was clearly nervous. He had a thin, reedy voice and tended to interject his phrases with an annoying number of "ums" and "ers." This did not make for a commanding lecture, but his address that evening was uncharacteristically short and elegant, and exhaustive. He had prepared for every possible critique.

He began by reminding his (all-male) audience of the vast toll TB had taken on humanity: "If the importance of a disease for mankind is measured by the number of fatalities it causes, then tuberculosis must be considered much more important than the most feared infectious diseases, plague, cholera, and the like. One in seven human beings dies from tuberculosis."

Koch's speech was about to solve the mystery of a common global foe that had long dogged science.

"All these facts taken together," he concluded, "can lead to only one conclusion. That the bacilli which are present in the tuberculosis substances not only accompany the tuberculosis process but are the cause of it. In the bacilli we have, therefore, the actual infective cause of tuberculosis."

Matter-of-factly, Koch had identified one of humanity's greatest killers. It was a momentous scientific whodunit, solved.

There were no questions from the audience; there were no interruptions during this lecture. The medical men were spellbound, aware of the fact that they were witnessing scientific history. It was uncharacteristic for there to be no interruptions. New science was usually immediately challenged by rivals short of good ideas. Yet the audience at the Physiological Society of Berlin were so dumbstruck that they did not even applaud. Everyone in the lecture hall understood the enormity of what had just happened. Within days, it was front-page news around the world. Within weeks, Koch was a household name.

In the room that night was a twenty-eight-year-old dermatologist named Paul Ehrlich, whose greatest achievement was the discovery of Salvarsan, or Compound 606, the first "magic bullet" against syphilis. Ehrlich later recalled the evening as "the most important experience" of his scientific life, and as soon as the lecture was completed, he rushed home to his makeshift laboratory, where he spent the night developing a staining technique using dyes to stain bacteria so they become visible, for the tubercle bacillus.[35]

This new understanding—that TB was infectious, not hereditary—called for a new type of treatment. Koch also realized that antibodies could help destroy the bacteria and build up immunity.

Seventeen days later, on April 10, 1882, Koch published his lecture, "The Etiology, or Cause, of Tuberculosis," in the *Berlin Clinical Weekly*.[36] Though TB was no longer a mysterious disease for the scientific community, Koch's understanding of how the disease worked did not translate into the immediate saving of lives. A full ten years later, Mercy Brown was exhumed from her grave by her terrified neighbors and her heart removed from her corpse and burned.

The next twenty years were a golden age of medical science, an extraordinary period setting in motion one of its most glorious eras. The miasmatic theory, eventually given up by scientists and physicians after 1880, was replaced by the germ theory of disease. Around the same time, the New England vampire scare started winding down, perhaps not coincidentally, as Robert Koch had identified the bacteria, taking the mystery away.

The vampire killers were finally found at the close of the nineteenth century.

With germ theory at its core, vaccines were developed to harmlessly simulate the disease, provoking the body to produce antibodies that inoculated against the deadly germs. This put in place a new branch of medicine we now know as immunology. Soon, pathogens were discovered for gonorrhea, bubonic plague, dysentery, tetanus, wound infections, and staph infections.

Unlike Semmelweis, who spent almost his entire professional life out of luck, these great scientists had nationalism, war, and chance all working in their favor. Chance, because they had access to technology such as the microscope, and they were better communicators than Semmelweis. They had one other advantage Semmelweis did not, which would prove crucial not in proving germ theory but in widely spreading the word: faster global communication.

Louis Pasteur became one of the greatest scientists of our time, revolutionized chemistry and biology, then founded microbiology. Koch went on to win a Nobel Prize in medicine. To this day, Joseph Lister is known as the Father of Antisepsis and Modern Surgery and is remembered—although not accurately—every time we rinse our mouths with a mouthwash named after him.

In the 1880s, Lister said he had heard of Semmelweis's work in the 1840s to 1860s. He generously credited Semmelweis, who had otherwise been forgotten, for the introduction of the principle of asepsis.[37] Based on the work of Louis Pasteur, Robert Koch, and Joseph Lister, the idea that Semmelweis did not find the words for—that germs caused disease and handwashing broke the chain of contamination—was finally established. By the mid-1890s, the medical community had dropped the term "consumption" in favor of the word "tuberculosis," thus linking the disease to the bacteria that caused it.

Semmelweis died without affirmation.

He had been right all along. Without a job, rejected and ridiculed, Semmelweis had refused to give up. He became obsessive—in every conversation Semmelweis turned to the topic of childbed fever. He sent his work to every notable obstetrician of the time.

The medical community considered it and unanimously rejected it.

With no alternative, he went on the offensive, grabbed a pen, and wrote a series of "open letters"—one of them ninety-two pages long—deriding his industry peers and former colleagues. He accused them of participating in "massacres" and called out as "murderers" all those who had failed to heed his rules.

He repeated his arguments, went again through the facts, prepared his rebuttals, and emphasized—as any good doctor must—the personal accountability of governments and obstetricians. He then took his case to those concerned: patients and the general public. Semmelweis had always refused to publish his results or deliver public lectures, yet fourteen years after his experiments at the maternity clinic in Vienna General Hospital, he relented and published his findings in a book entitled *The Etiology, Concept, and Prophylaxis of Childbed Fever*. In the preface he wrote, "By nature, I am averse to all polemics. . . . I believed that I could leave it to time to break a path for the truth. However, for thirteen years, my expectations have not been fulfilled. . . . Fate has chosen me as a representative of truths. . . . It is my inescapable obligation to support them. . . . I feel that it would be a sin to keep silent."[38]

It was part rambling history of his findings and part instruction manual for hospital hygiene. The second half of the book was, disturbingly for his peers, a vicious rant against those who doubted him. His book failed commercially, and he grew increasingly unstable, to the point that he would randomly accost young couples in the street, begging them to make sure their doctor washed his hands if they ever had a child.

He interpreted calls for proof by his colleagues as a personal insult and responded rudely, writing to one obstetrician in Vienna, "You, Herr Professor, have been a partner in this massacre." To another, "Should you, Herr Hofrath, without having disproved my doctrine, continue to train your pupils [against it], I declare before God and the world that you are a murderer and the 'History of Childbed Fever' would not be unjust to you if it memorialized you as a medical Nero."[39] Ignaz Semmelweis's story is a tragic case of science denialism, still common today, and is known summarily as the "Semmelweis reflex" or "Semmelweis effect," describing the reflex-like tendency to reject new evidence or knowledge that contradicts established norms, beliefs, or paradigms.

Human beings like information to be consistent with our belief systems, however faulty our beliefs may be. When dissonant information is presented, discrediting the facts or the fact-speaker is the least unsettling way to handle the challenge posed by the new information that is not aligned with the majority's worldview. We have seen it repeatedly, as climate-change denialism, HIV denialism, and vaccination denialism.

In 1865—just as Pasteur was conducting his silkworm experiments and Lister was operating on the broken leg of an eleven-year-old boy—Semmelweis was committed to a mental asylum. Expressing concern over his spiraling mental health, his wife and family convinced him to travel to a spa in Gräfenberg in southern Germany to undergo water treatments.[40] At this point, Semmelweis's tragic story turns sinister. His family had used subterfuge to have him committed. Committal required the signatures of three doctors. Semmelweis's wife, Maria, contacted Lajos Markusovszky, his colleague and closest friend from his days as a medical student, who asked a pediatrician to examine him. The pediatrician concluded that Semmelweis was insane. Two other physicians, neither of whom had examined Semmelweis, also signed commitment papers.

Semmelweis was taken by overnight train to Vienna after being led to believe that he was on the way to Gräfenberg. He was met at the station on August 7 by Markusovszky, who told Semmelweis he wanted to show him his clinic in Lazarettgasse. Once inside the asylum, Semmelweis was greeted by burly orderlies bearing a straitjacket.

He had been duped.

Six days later, on the evening of August 13, 1865, Dr. Ignaz Fülöp Semmelweis was pronounced dead. No priest was called to administer his last rites. There is no record of what happened to him during the days he spent at the asylum, but a postmortem report leaves little to the imagination: he was beaten by his attendants, trampled, placed in a straitjacket, and left to die of his injuries.

An autopsy was performed on his body in the same morgue in which he himself had conducted so many postmortem examinations of women who had died of childbed fever. Based on the autopsy report, he had probably been beaten twice, with both of his arms broken, and then secured in a straitjacket. He had been strapped to a bed. By the time the straps were removed, both of his forearms had become gangrenous.

Thanks to modern medicine, we now know that Semmelweis died of sepsis, a potentially fatal complication of an infection in the bloodstream—basically, the same disease he fought so hard to prevent in those women who died from childbed fever. The entry point of the infection could have been a wound in the middle finger of Semmelweis's right hand, acquired during his beatings.

He was forty-seven years old.

On August 15, he was buried in Vienna. Not a single member of his family was present, nor a single colleague.[41] Almost no one in the medical community acknowledged his passing: "One said nothing of Semmelweis, it was as though one was ashamed of his memory."[42] In 1891, his remains were moved to Budapest, and once again on October 11, 1964, to the courtyard of his family house in Tabán, where he had been born.

---•---

CHAPTER 3

THE MAN PROBLEM

t is hard to imagine America as a nation dealing with an explosion of tuberculosis. The English writer Charles Dickens dubbed America a moist "nation of spitters."[1] He arrived at Boston Harbor in 1842, as a thirty-year-old literary celebrity, where he was repulsed by Americans' table manners and the tobacco expectoration everywhere he looked. After visiting the US Congress in 1842, he wrote in his "American Notes for General Circulation" that Washington, DC, was "the head-quarters of tobacco-tinctured saliva. . . . Both houses are handsomely carpeted; but the state to which these carpets are reduced by the universal disregard of the spittoon . . . and the extraordinary improvements on the pattern which are squirted and dabbled upon in every direction . . . do not admit of being described," Dickens wrote, appalled.

"I will merely observe, that I strongly recommend all strangers not to look at the floor; and if they happen to drop anything, though it be their purse, not to pick it up with an ungloved hand on any account."

This changed once germ theory was widely accepted.

The idea of germs infiltrated the American imagination. State governments spent aggressively on public health campaigns, where doctors advised a combination of fresh air, clean water, healthy food, and safe medicine to cure tuberculosis.

It is around this time that Americans realized they had a "man problem."

In the new germ-conscious age, spitting became taboo. Except that half the population seemed not to have gotten the message, despite newspapers condemning habitual spitters and encouraging citizens to spread the antispitting gospel.

The most prominent government strategy was adopted by America's most densely populated city—New York—which resorted to legislative prohibition, passing the nation's first spitting ban and encouraging New Yorkers to cover their coughs and sneezes. In 1889, New York City began America's first campaign to control tuberculosis when a group of prominent doctors in New York presented the city's health department with a report that linked TB to spitting, coughing, and sneezing.

Pulmonary tuberculosis (the kind that infects the lungs) alone caused 237 deaths per 100,000 people. In 1900, it was estimated that the death rate for TB for white Americans was between 190 and 200 per 100,000. Among black Americans, the comparable figure was 400 deaths per 100,000. Nationwide, approximately 150,000 Americans died from TB each year, and a million more were infected. A century later, thanks to sustained public health efforts, this had fallen to less than 1 death per 100,000 people.[2] The drastic drop in number of deaths was brought on by three control measures: intensive screening among at-risk populations, such as the poor and the homeless; better training of staff and availability of facilities to ensure that patients completed therapy; and, if necessary, detention of individuals who did not take their medications.[3] The measures would make the twentieth century the turning point in the war against consumption.

Physicians recommended a series of measures to stop the spread of TB, and the New York City Health Department, headed by Hermann M. Biggs from 1892 to 1901, responded to this by distributing a leaflet of health-conscious behaviors.[4]

The city implored New Yorkers to sleep separately from TB patients and to separate their clothing, and the most significant rule was to forbid "persons suspected to have consumption to spit on the floor or on cloths unless the latter be immediately burned."[5] The 1889 leaflet was the first attempt to explicitly connect spitting to the transmission of tuberculosis and in turn promote certain social expectations of hygiene. Seven years later, in 1896, New York City became the first American metropolis to ban spitting altogether. The city put up antispitting notices. It was now punishable to spit on sidewalks, in public buildings, on public transit, and "other spitting hot spots," giving officials the ability to slap wayward spitters with a fine or a jail sentence. From the government's perspective, the well-being of society superseded the right of any individual to indiscriminately spit.

New York followed its strong words with actions: the city conducted "dragnets," or police raids, that arrested masses of spitters in a single day and then publicized the arrests.

None of it made a difference.

Spitting remained a ubiquitous habit that, depending on gender, Americans either enjoyed or put up with.

The New York Department of Health was at the start of a decades-long process of changing the behavior of American men by encouraging them to think of spitting as a public health threat. Brooklyn, which passed an ordinance quickly after New York City, called on local volunteer organizations to help spread the word.

The anti-TB crusade brought together natural allies: the New York City Health Department, the National Tuberculosis Association in Brooklyn and New York City, and the Women's Health Protective Association.

Bringing in women to craft slogans was a smart choice.

Behavior science shows that laws plus awareness plus public shaming is a recipe for behavior change. American women still did not have the right to vote, but they were an influential voice of reason and actively fought for years to improve public health.

Among the first decisions made by this group of women was to drop the word "expectorate" on notices in favor of "spit." Meeting minutes reveal how they debated over a simple yet effective message. The phrase "Do not spit on the floor of this car" was proposed and later opposed because women argued it wasn't foolproof: men would simply be encouraged to spit on walls and windows. After some discussion, the phrase "spitting positively forbidden" became the winning catchphrase for the women's campaign. They also "generated other antispitting slogans such as 'Spitting Is Dangerous, Indecent, and Against the Law,' 'Beware the Careless Spitter,' and 'No Spit, No Consumption.' They made posters decrying spitting . . . and reminding people of the ban. Members of the public were encouraged to confront defiant spitters or, at the very least," reproach them by staring the spitters into shame.[6] Soon, health departments throughout the United States followed New York's lead. Over the next fifteen years, almost 150 other US cities banned public spitting.

By now, there was enough data to profile the offender: he was almost universally male.

The antispitting crusaders found that men from all social classes, ethnic backgrounds, and professions spat more often than women. As cities enforced their new ordinances, they fined and arrested wage laborers, professors, attorneys, and even mayors. Following a Pittsburgh dragnet in 1907, reporters noted that the only distinguishing feature of the one hundred arrested spitters was their diversity: "There was no discrimination as to race, colour, creed, or station in life. . . . The labourer rubbed elbows with the business man, and the merchant was followed by an alien or a negro."[7]

Soon, municipal authorities noticed that the spitting ban was difficult to enforce. A habit so ingrained could not be corrected with an ad campaign alone. So, cities stationed police officers on every public conveyance and within every public building, and to mitigate gaps in enforcement, civilians were encouraged, even expected, to stand up to spitters.

By now, the constant barrage of behavior-change messages had begun to anger some men. In one extreme example, an arresting officer in Minnesota so infuriated a group of spitters that they turned on him and beat him until his "head [was] broken, two of his ribs [were] fractured, and his body [was] seriously bruised."[8] Many police officers concluded that the antispitting campaign was simply not worth the trouble. Besides, most police officers, also men, didn't see any harm in spitting.

A thesis on the antispitting movement by Patrick J. O'Connor, a student at the University of Montana–Missoula, quoted a Buffalo police officer who argued that "it's a pretty hard thing to arrest a man merely for spitting on the floor. . . . I don't see any harm about it, unless a feller does it on a man's shoes."

During the same week, a reporter witnessed another officer spitting on a streetcar while he was supposed to be on patrol to prevent the activity.

Magistrates also resisted enforcing antispitting ordinances. Judges, again all men, regularly released spitters without punishment. Spitting had become so much of a reflex that most men, even after all the campaigns, did not realize that they were spitting. When confronted with their actions, they flatly denied that they were spitters moments after splattering the street.

Frustrated, the government tried a different tack: they declared that a good male citizen should prioritize public health over personal comfort and set an example for others by not spitting. A "manly man" would not spit or let anyone else spit, they said.

They encouraged men to police each other, and every woman was encouraged to "slowly rise from her seat and draw her skirts carefully about her feet, meanwhile transfixing the offender with a hard-boiled eye, and then reseat herself with equal care." Basically, the government asked women to give erring men the stink-eye.

Still, nothing happened.

The spitting continued unabated. Spit adorned city sidewalks, gathered in women's dresses, and entered homes on the soles of men's shoes. And tuberculosis thrived as bacteria-infected sputum spread to every corner of the city. TB was killing one in seven Americans at this point.[9] As if in mockery of city ordinances, men would spit on posters ordering them not to. The government went back to the drawing board and came up with a new strategy, a tailor-made antispitting message for each socioeconomic group.

In the new message, immigrants and members of the working class—the groups with the highest risk of contracting tuberculosis—were asked to abstain from spitting, as it could spread the disease. The middle class was told to stop because they served as an example to their social "inferiors." The upper class was told it was their responsibility to help quell the disease but also to promote middle-class values and better hygiene practices.

By the turn of the century, Koch's linking of tuberculosis to a bacterium had opened the door for mass public health campaigns. Whether they were riding in streetcars, entering public buildings, or, as the scope of ordinances expanded, walking on sidewalks, the public was constantly reminded not to spit. Citizens could not escape the antispitting messages, and the traditional expectation of women as housekeepers was expanded to the entire city, with women being seen as "municipal housekeepers."[10] A Sterling, Kansas, woman's 1904 poem illustrates the ubiquity of notices and their effect on a young spitter in her town, which had recently passed an ordinance of its own:

> *The shades of night were falling fast*
> *As through a Kansas city passed*
> *A youth who saw, all fresh and nice,*
> *A poster with this strange device—*
> *Please do not spit on the sidewalks.*
> *His brow was sad; and in his cheek*
> *A quid so big he scarce could speak;*
> *It seemed to be on ev'ry tongue,—*
> *On ev'ry passing breeze 'twas flung,*
> *Please do not spit on the sidewalks.*

The omnipresent, incrementally assertive antispitting campaign was still, however, largely ineffectual. If anything, it annoyed many men, who spat with ever greater determination.

In 1895, a Pennsylvania doctor named Elmer B. Borland presented a paper about the dangers of spitting to the Allegheny

County Medical Society. Like many formally trained physicians, Borland had become convinced that "restriction and regulation of the spitting habit" was necessary if they were to control the spiraling TB epidemic.[11] Borland made a convincing argument.

> Writing about the speech several years later in the *Journal of the American Medical Association*, Borland recalled that "nine of the ten members who took part in the discussion agreed that restriction and regulation were needed." Of that group, however, six thought any form of regulation impractical. They believed passage of such regulations would be difficult, if not impossible, and lamented that "women can, but men can not, change their filthy spitting habit." Borland disagreed, arguing that "most men had the natural instinct of cleanliness and could be educated up to this level with women." Those who could not—"the ignorant, unteachable, and vicious"—must be controlled anyway, for the tragedy of tuberculosis demanded it.[12]

At the 1901 British Congress of Tuberculosis, after being shamed for a few years, men turned the applecart over. The congress determined that the best way to fix the problem of TB was not to try to correct men's spitting habits but to adjust women's hemlines.

They went after the low-hanging skirt.

Men argued that women were to blame for wearing clothes that brushed the pavements, picking up the germs men spat out.

The antispitting campaigns, so far, had relied on the assumption that reform was necessary to "protect women," because their long dresses were prone to gather spit from floors, stairs, or sidewalks. Women represented the most obvious victims of indiscriminate spitting. The onus for preventing the spread of germs was on women since they were the ones who cleaned their homes and prepared food. Since they were already cleaning up after men, why not make them take the extra step of adjusting their dresses?

Some women protested at the one-sidedness of being held responsible for the consequences of men's nasty habits. In 1903, at a public meeting on expanding the scope of the antispitting law in Washington, Ellen Spencer Mussey, a lawyer and pioneer in women's rights advocacy, got up to speak on behalf of "7,000 of her sex" who were "unanimously in favor of restrictions in the habit of spitting upon the public streets of the city." She also connected it to children's welfare, as "those playing on the sidewalks in front of their homes" were often "exposed to the disease germs from sputum."

But there were plenty of dismal male voices to shout down Mussey's opinions. Dr. Charles Allen, an opponent of the antispitting campaign, called it a ridiculous crusade against men before he too identified the real culprit: ladies in trailing skirts.

Such fashions, and the women who wore them, acted as "breeders of disease," and rather than regulating men's behaviors for the convenience of fashion, Dr. Allen argued women should curtail their dresses and accommodate spitters.

In a world ruled by men, of course, this argument found plenty of takers. Large-scale American and public health campaigns started targeting women's fashion. Doctors began to decry long, trailing skirts as culprits of disease.

Men took this argument seriously enough to propose legislation enforcing it. They even came up with a catchy name for the skirt that swept the floor: the septic skirt.

Since the 1880s, women had tried to reform their clothing, especially as they moved toward careers in sports and entertainment, but they were unsuccessful until men were prohibited from spitting.

The O'Connor paper, on the American antispitting campaign between 1896 and 1910, states that "a writer identifying himself as *Libertas* wrote to the *Brooklyn Daily Eagle* and accused anti-spitters of sending men to jail because "the dress of the wife of [a member] of the Department of Health . . . was soiled by contact with the street."

In Columbus, Ohio, a city councilor proposed a companion ordinance to antispitting that would require women to wear dresses "at least 3 inches from the ground."

In 1900, the New York magazine *Puck* featured a freakish cartoon on its cover—*The Trailing Skirt: Death Loves a Shining Mark*.[13] It showed a maid shaking off clouds of germs from her deadly skirt and demonized it further by showing angelic-looking children in the background as clouds of "consumption," "influenza," and "typhoid" rose from it. A skeleton holding a scythe, death itself, looming right behind the maid, rammed home the message: the skirt was the killer.

Many women responded to the fear-mongering chorus and shortened their skirts so they no longer swept the streets. The rising hemline, often considered to be a sign of sexual freedom, began as a consequence of germ theory and male inconsideration.

A small group of American women led by actress Bertha Welby had already been promoting short skirts. Their group was called the Rainy Day Club, since the women's objection to the sweeping skirts was that they caught germs, dust, and rain.

It was set up in 1896, the same year New York City passed prohibitive legislation banning spitting. The club members were called Rainy Daisies and were initially ridiculed by the public. However, with the doctors' endorsements, the merits of the Rainy

Daisies' skirts were accepted, and manufactures began making shorter skirts.[14]

As women's hemlines rose a few inches at the beginning of the 1900s, shoes became an important feature of women's fashion. Corsets came under attack too, as they were believed to exacerbate tuberculosis. Malleable as ever, women moved to "health corsets," made with elastic fabric that alleviated pressure on the ribs.

TB would impact male fashion too.

Many men were guilty of sporting a dust trap right under their noses: their beards. By the 1900s, beards and mustaches were deemed dangerous, thanks to the germ theory. "There is no way of computing the number of bacteria and noxious germs that may lurk in the Amazonian jungles of a well-whiskered face, but their number must be legion," Edwin F. Bowers, an American doctor known for pioneering reflexology, wrote in a 1916 issue of *McClure's Magazine*.[15] "Measles, scarlet fever, diphtheria, tuberculosis, whooping cough, common and uncommon colds, and a host of other infectious diseases can be, and undoubtedly are, transmitted via the whisker route." By the time Bowers penned his spirited essay, facial hair had largely disappeared from the faces of American men, especially surgeons and physicians, who adopted the clean-shaven look to be more hygienic when caring for patients.

Before Pasteur and Koch's research, a beard was thought to possess qualities that positioned it as a kind of health shield for the face. In 1881, an article in *St. James Magazine*, titled "Beards," written by Dr. Tom Robinson, an English physician, "encouraged men to grow facial hair to help prevent illness. According to Robinson, who drew on medical literature dating back to the Renaissance . . . medical conditions such as loose and sore teeth, nasal catarrh . . .

and facial neuralgia . . . could all be prevented."[16] The piece goes on to say, "Soldiers with facial hair were less likely to be admitted to hospital with respiratory ailments such as bronchitis because it was believed that the hair could sift out harmful particles in the air."

New research showed that beards could indeed harbor bacteria linked to the spread of infectious diseases: spittle caught in the hairs of the beard could contain tuberculosis. To avoid germs men were encouraged to shave regularly. Eventually, hospitals in Britain banned beards altogether, and it fell to nurses to remove their patients' facial hair as part of their health-care duties.

Seeing a new demand for razors, a salesman called King Gillette marketed a unique invention that revolutionized the shaving industry. In 1903, an editorial, "Passing of the Beard," ran in *Harper's Weekly*.

It noted nostalgically that the beard had become popular as a tool that covered deformities on faces, kept throats warm, and lastly, purified the air entering their mouths but ended: "Now that consumption is no longer consumption, but tuberculosis, and is not hereditary but infectious . . . the theory of science is that the beard is infected with the germs of tuberculosis." Ultimately, the clean-shaven look became a symbol of the new middle-class man during a period *Harper's Weekly* labeled "the revolt against the whisker."

While it changed fashion and ushered in new grooming styles, the fear of TB did not put an end to spitting. The laws were still difficult to implement, and police officers were baffled when they confronted a spitter who brazenly denied it.

Spitters, when confronted by police officials, would often deny having spat at all. For example, during his arrest for spitting on Brooklyn's Fifth Avenue elevated car in 1901, William McDonald told the arresting officer that "he really had no idea that he had been spitting in the car." To make men such as McDonald entirely conscious of their behavior and then to expect him to hold his spit until he found a handkerchief, or a bathroom, seemed a herculean task.

Even their harshest derision did not bring about behavioral change in men.

In response, medical and municipal authorities devised a handful of strategies that they hoped would end spitting once and for all. The "dragnets" were still being conducted, and now municipal authorities started publicizing the arrests. They were ordered to arrest each spitter and immediately bring him to the city's police court, where he was quickly tried, fined, and released.

A second and reasonably successful strategy came from the Cook County, Illinois, League of Women's Clubs, who recommended providing sand to streetcar conductors with which they could "cover the objectionable spots on streetcar floors." It was the next best solution, given that they could not get men to stop spitting.

In 1910, St. Louis physician Robert Newton argued that since 1896, a total of 2,513 spitters had been arrested in New York, but only 908 spitters faced similar consequences throughout the rest of the country. He was presenting the data before the National Association for the Study and Prevention of Tuberculosis. Considering that approximately 25 million Americans lived in communities with antispitting health campaigns, Newton believed the total of 3,421 arrests ("undoubtedly all males," he noted) represented "a failure to enforce the laws." Further, of those 3,421, only 2,912 were convicted, with fines averaging only about $1.40, the equivalent of around $27 in today's currency.

The most practical strategy, given how unpliable men were, came when the antituberculosis campaign accessorized itself.

Enter the spittoon, a fabulous little invention that allowed men to chew tobacco and then fling the brownish spit into a little brass bucket. The spittoon allowed men to pretty much spit wherever and whenever they needed to. Soon, spittoons, personal cuspidors, or pocket flasks became manly accessories. S. Adolphus Knopf, an early TB specialist who practiced medicine in New York, hoped that they would allow the spitter to continue his disgusting habit without soiling public space or spreading disease.[17] The flasks were marketed specifically to tuberculosis patients, with Kny-Scheerer Company, a New York–based manufacture of medical instruments, offering discounts to dealers for "quantity orders" from sanatoriums and hospitals.

Instead of fining or dragnetting people, health authorities started giving the spitters some options: do it in the toilet, in a handkerchief, or in a spittoon. Many states saw a proliferation of brass spittoons that were strategically placed in public places that were spitting hotspots. Personal hand-size spittoons were also marketed to men who wanted to be polite while doing this. Spittoons could be found in offices, hotels, bars, and public buildings. The government updated their advisories: men were now urged to shave their beards and carry pocket spittoons. Women were urged to stop wearing trailing dresses, and children were taught to keep their faces, hands, and fingernails clean and "cough and sneeze in your elbows please."[18] Did the measures championed by the US improve mortality rates of TB, influenza, pneumonia, and other airborne illnesses rising from the cloud of the trailing skirt?

Yes, indeed.[19] Between 1900 and 1904, tuberculosis was causing 256 deaths per 100,000 people in New York City. By the 1940s, this number had been reduced to 40 per 100,000.

The US Centers for Disease Control and Prevention (CDC) still finds itself needing to remind Americans of the benefits of frequent handwashing and masking coughs and sneezes to prevent the spread of germs.

In *The Gospel of Germs*, Nancy Tomes offers a gripping social history of how the awareness of how germs spread gave rise to new social habits and customs. People learned to shield their sneezes and coughs, rejected handshaking, and frowned upon kissing someone else's baby.[20] Domestic awareness of hygiene radiated outward as well: we have anti-TB reformers to thank for higher sanitary standards in hotels, railway cars, and movie theaters, which were remodeled with easily cleanable tiles in place of the old-world rugs and heavy curtains that were dust and germ traps.

Linens were changed daily in hotels; it is because of the anti-TB movement that you get your own bar of soap, a fresh towel, and clean sheets.

CHAPTER 4

---◆---

THE DOCTOR FROM
SOUTHSEA

Doctors have an enduring love affair with the private detective Sherlock Holmes. Long before Arthur Conan Doyle created Holmes, he was an ordinary British physician with a failing private practice in Southsea, along the south coast of England.

He had trained at the University of Edinburgh Medical School as a physician and received a bachelor of medicine and master of surgery qualifications from the University of Edinburgh in 1881 and an MD in 1885.[1] There, Doyle was known for his curiosity. As a twenty-year-old second-year medical student, he published his first academic paper, titled "Gelsemium as a Poison," in the *British Medical Journal* on September 20, 1879.[2] To write the paper, he ingested the poison to see how it could be used to treat neuropathic (nerve) pain. He self-administered the poison at increasing doses for seven days, at the same time each day. At low doses he observed that twenty minutes after ingesting the poison, he experienced extreme "giddiness." As he increased the dosage, he noticed that the giddiness was lessened, but he had vision problems. At an even higher dosage, he had headaches and diarrhea. This is where most would have stopped, but not Doyle. He pushed on toward a dosage high enough to cause "persistent and prostrating" diarrhea, headache, and weak pulse. He signed off a letter describing the experiment so clinically and dispassionately, it is easy to imagine that Holmes himself might be writing:

> I feel convinced that I could have taken as much as half an ounce of the tincture, had it not been for the extreme diarrhoea it brought on.
> —Believe me, yours sincerely,
> A. C. D.
> Clifton House, Aston Road, Birmingham.

Doyle's drug-dabbling ways made for enthralling stories that were inspired by medicines, his mentors, his real patients, and his friends from medical school. After graduating, Doyle attempted to set up a private practice, but it didn't thrive.

In any case, his true passion was writing.

Since the patients were few, he took to writing short stories in his unoccupied time. In his autobiography, he wrote, "Every morning I walked from the lodgings, at Montague Place, reached my consulting-room at ten and sat there until three or four, with never a ring to disturb my serenity. Could better conditions for reflection be found? It was ideal, and so long as I was thoroughly unsuccessful in my professional venture there was every chance of improvement in my literary prospects."[3] *A Study in Scarlet*—in which the detectives named Sherlock Holmes and Dr. Watson make their first appearance—was published in 1887.

While Doyle is popularly known for his novels, he was also a sleuth in his own profession. He believed in the new age of scientific medicine, as is evident in his writing, where he used new science to solve everyday problems and mysteries. Before he wrote Sherlock, Doyle would write essays explaining new, evolving medicine to laypeople. He was an important translator for the general public of the cutting-edge science doctors like Robert Koch, Joseph Lister, and Louis Pasteur were practicing.

As Doyle was sitting down in his not-so-popular clinic to write medical mysteries, Robert Koch was making headlines. By 1890, Koch had discovered the agent that caused cholera, tuberculosis, and anthrax. His postulates had become an accepted scientific framework to prove that a particular microbe causes a specific infectious disease, and he had revolutionized medicine.

Now, he was getting ready for an even more momentous announcement.

On August 6, 1890, around six thousand physicians—the eminences of medicine from around the world—were gathered at the Tenth International Medical Congress in Berlin. The biggest star in this gathering was, of course, Robert Koch. It was a blistering day in Berlin, but the physicians seated in the stifling hot auditorium were not to be disappointed.

Koch announced that he had a "remedy" for tuberculosis.

In a world connected by telegraphs and newspapers—as well as a world in which tuberculosis was a leading cause of death and illness—his announcement was front-page news. Koch was the hero of the German Empire and the object of adulation throughout Europe. He did not want to be scooped again by Pasteur in finding a cure for TB. Koch had closed himself in his lab and secretly developed a "plasma" he called tuberculin and claimed that it cured TB. Koch told the newspaper that he had found *das heilmittel*, German for "the remedy," and arranged for a demonstration on November 17.[4] Doyle was following these developments keenly from his perch in Southsea. Intrigued by the reports of the impending demonstration, he decided he wanted to witness history being made. He pitched a story idea to an editor of a London newspaper called the *Review of Reviews* and dashed to Berlin to attend the November lecture.

Doyle arrived in Berlin on a Sunday. The Koch lecture was the most anticipated event of the conference, and he could not secure the golden ticket. He went to the British embassy in Berlin, hoping the ambassador would help him. He had no luck.

Doyle next appeared, unannounced, at Koch's home. Still, no luck.

Koch's butler told Doyle that the professor was unavailable. The next morning, Doyle turned up at the lecture hall and tried to bribe a guard and gain entry. The lecture hall was packed, the guard refused, and Doyle later recounted, "To the Englishman in Berlin, and indeed to the German also, it is at present very much easier to see the bacillus of Koch than to catch even the most fleeting glimpse of its discoverer."

Eventually, even though he could not get a seat, an American physician from Detroit named Henry Hartz offered to share his notes from the lecture. Doyle got along with Hartz well enough for Hartz to allow him to make his own copy. After Doyle had carefully read the notes, the two physicians visited the wards where patients had been treated with tuberculin.

Doyle tried one last time to meet Dr. Koch in his laboratory but was denied an audience. Doyle was skeptical of the remedy. He discovered that Koch violated his own principles—the postulates—when he worked in secret and refused to disclose his methods.

The more Doyle investigated Koch's discovery, the more his claims of a remedy fell apart. Doyle looked at the clinical data, did the math, and realized Koch's theory did not stand up to scrutiny.

Once you eliminate the impossible, whatever remains, no matter how improbable, must be the truth, as Holmes would later say.

The truth, according to Doyle, was that Koch was lying. His first dispatch, a letter to the *Daily Telegraph* published on November 20, 1890, under the title "The Consumption Cure," said, "Great as is Koch's discovery, there can be no question that our knowledge of it is still very incomplete, and that it leaves large issues open to questions."

"The whole thing was experimental and premature," he concluded. On his return to England, he published a scathing four-thousand-word report on Koch's cure, essentially calling it a cruel hoax. The *Review of Reviews* ran it in December of that year. While many rejoiced the conquest of tuberculosis, Doyle argued that "Koch's lymph" might remove traces of the diseased tissue, but it left deadly germs "deep in the invaded country."

Its real value, Doyle asserted, was as "an admirable aid to diagnosis," in that a "single injection" would help doctors decide definitively whether a patient was "in any way tuberculous."[5] But as for the cure itself, he said, "It is as if a man whose house was infested with rats were to remove the marks of the creatures every morning and expect in that way to get rid of them. . . . Unfortunately, it is evident that the system soon establishes a tolerance to the injected fluid, so that the time must apparently come when the continually renewed tubercle tissue will refuse to respond to the remedy."[6] Doyle was correct in his conclusions. Koch's new treatment temporarily suppressed symptoms, and then the disease got worse. Koch spent several months defending the curative properties of tuberculin. But when his patients started failing, he could no longer defend it.

In early 1891, after several highly publicized treatment failures and a few deaths associated with the administration of the so-called curative medication, Koch publicly retracted his earlier announcement. The lymph, he explained, was an excellent means of diagnosing tuberculosis, but an actual cure for the White Plague was nowhere in sight.

It is difficult not to be impressed by Doyle's far-reaching deductions, especially since it took Koch, one of the most illustrious medical detectives in the world, many more months to realize his error.[7] Doyle achieved another insight long before antibiotics had been invented: that bacteria would develop resistance to treatments. All along, Doyle had been writing as well. He published "A Scandal in Bohemia," the first short story featuring literature's most famous detective, Sherlock Holmes, in 1891. Doyle eventually decided to abandon his failing practice in Southsea and move to London, where he started writing the Sherlock Holmes stories. He was immediately successful, and money started to pour in such that he could make writing his primary activity.

By 1893, Doyle was tired of Holmes and thought the character "tended to obscure" his higher work. In "The Final Problem," Holmes falls to his death over the Reichenbach Falls while fighting his archenemy, Professor Moriarty.

England mourned. His fans wore black badges on their sleeves.

The public outcry was so great that Doyle resurrected the detective.

He continued his medical practice for another decade and in 1900 volunteered to serve as a doctor in a military hospital during the Boer War. He was a man with a restlessly inquiring mind and strong opinions, not all backed by good science or good sense.

His enthusiastic spiritualism seems impractical today, though Doyle made a plausible psychological connection between the trauma experienced by the survivors of World War I and their grieving families and the rise of spiritualist beliefs. He also defended the British Empire's role in South Africa, despite the appalling cruelty inflicted in its name. During the Boer War, British troops rounded up tens of thousands of Dutch-speaking women, children, and elderly people, along with their black servants, and sent them to concentration camps. The death rate was catastrophic. "160,000 Boers were incarcerated, 28,000 died, more than 22,000 of them children." Angered by charges that the British committed atrocities during the Boer War, Doyle wrote, in one week, a sixty-thousand-word pamphlet in rebuttal.[8] This pamphlet, defending British actions in South Africa—rather than his literary achievements—got him knighted.

The doctor from Southsea became Sir Arthur Conan Doyle, which is how he is known today.

The character of Sherlock Holmes, though, emerged from good science and sense. The novels were based on one of Doyle's professors and mentors at Edinburgh, Dr. Joseph Bell. Bell was renowned for his extraordinary observational abilities. Doyle first met Bell in 1877 when he was a medical student. He had served as a clerk for Bell and spent a great deal of time observing his deductive abilities.

In many ways, Doyle was Dr. Watson to Bell's Sherlock Holmes.

Bell could tell from the tattoos of sailors where they had sailed, could discern a man's origin from his accent, and could tell the profession of a patient from glancing at their hands. He famously concluded that one man was an alcoholic by observing that he habitually carried a flask in the inside breast pocket of his coat. He is reported to have noted that another man was a cobbler by seeing that the inside of the knee of the man's trousers was worn in a particular way.[9] Doyle later recollected one example of Bell's exceptional use of science for deductive reasoning when Bell observed a patient that he had never spoken to or met before: "Well, my man," Bell said, after a quick glance at the patient, "you've served in the army."

"Aye, sir," the patient replied.

"Not long discharged?"

"No, sir."

"A Highland regiment?"

"Aye, sir."

"A non-com officer?"

"Aye, sir."

"Stationed at Barbados?"

"Aye, sir."

Bell turned to his bewildered students. "You see, gentlemen," he explained, "the man was a respectful man but did not remove his hat. They do not in the army, but he would have learned civilian's ways had he been long discharged. He has an air of authority, and he is obviously Scottish. As to Barbados, his complaint is elephantiasis, which is West Indian and not British, and the Scottish regiments are at present in that particular island."[10] Within medical circles, this story of Bell's diagnosis is legendary. That's not where the resemblance ends. Joseph Bell is reported to have often worn a long coat and a deerstalker hat. Doyle once wrote to Bell thanking him and acknowledging him for his influence in the creation of his most famous character: "It is most certainly to you that I owe Sherlock Holmes. . . . Round the centre of deduction and inference and observation which I have heard you inculcate, I have tried to build up a man who pushed the thing as far as it would go—further occasionally—and I am so glad that the result has satisfied you."

Through his novels, Doyle played a huge role in making cutting-edge science available to the general public. His novels discreetly popularized contemporary scientific thinking and approaches. In his fiction and nonfiction, he was always a careful science reporter in the golden era of science.

And in Sherlock Holmes's amiable sidekick, Dr. John H. Watson, Doyle added a character who had experience—military, medical, and political—of another of Britain's colonies. Watson had served as a military surgeon, like Doyle himself, not in South Africa but in the jewel of Britain's imperial crown, India.

It is to India that the story of tuberculosis also turns.

Not that consumptive deaths disappeared from Europe and America in the twentieth century. Orwell and Kafka were victims of tuberculosis, as were Eleanor Roosevelt, Polish composer Frédéric Chopin, English novelist Jane Austen, and American essayist and philosopher Henry David Thoreau. All of the Brontë sisters—Charlotte, Elizabeth, Emily, and Anne—died from various forms of tuberculosis between September 1848 and May 1855. English poet John Keats's entire family died from TB, and he composed "Ode to a Nightingale" six months after his brother's death from the illness. He referred to it as his "family disease" and was twenty-five when he succumbed to it too.

Thanks to relentless heartache, the lore around TB found an unlikely ally: art. It became, counterintuitively, known as a "romantic malady," inspiring operas such as *La traviata* (on which the film

Moulin Rouge is based) and becoming a steady feature in several Dickensian novels, such as *Dombey and Son*. In his third novel, *Nicholas Nickleby* (1839), Dickens writes about the suffering of TB patients almost as if they are being cleansed by consumption:

> There is a dread disease which so prepares its victim, as it were, for death; which so refines it of its grosser aspect, and throws around familiar looks unearthly indications of the coming change; a dread disease, in which the struggle between soul and body is so gradual, quiet, and solemn, and the result so sure, that day by day, and grain by grain, the mortal part wastes and withers away, so that the spirit grows light and sanguine with its lightening load, and, feeling immortality at hand, deems it but a new term of mortal life; a disease in which death and life are so strangely blended, that death takes the glow and hue of life, and life the gaunt and grisly form of death; a disease which medicine never cured, wealth never warded off, or poverty could boast exemption from; which sometimes moves in giant strides, and sometimes at a tardy sluggish pace, but, slow or quick, is ever sure and certain.[11]

This view of TB—as mysterious, romantic malady—changed once slum clearances, municipal sewage systems, and safe and sterile drinking water were provided to urban centers in the US and Europe. Access to modern medicine became a reality, and tuberculosis was never again considered the captain of the men of death.

PART II

CHAPTER 5

———◆———

INSIDE BUILDING
NUMBER 10

Mumbai is one of India's largest cities, with a population of more than twenty million people. People have lived here since at least the Pleistocene era, and all the European adventurers found their way to Mumbai, thanks to its many natural bays on the Arabian Sea, beginning with the Portuguese in 1534.

The city has more millionaires and billionaires than any other in India. It also has more tuberculosis than any other city in India. Any attempt to understand the global TB epidemic must travel through Mumbai, the epicenter of the crisis.

Like all great cities of the postindustrial world, Mumbai is a fevered dream. It is ancient, it is modern, and it is complicated.

Mumbai, like India, lives in several centuries at the same time. In 2006, Anthony Bourdain shot season 2 of *No Reservations* in India. The episode began with Bourdain saying, "To be in India, anywhere in India, is to risk being endlessly enchanted and repelled, until your senses want to shut down."

That is India's mythology—rich, fanciful, and vast.

Over centuries, migrants and invaders came here looking for home and, by a process of synthesis and absorption, made it what it is. Being one of the oldest civilizations in the world, India is the birthplace of four existing religions—Hinduism, Buddhism, Jainism, and Sikhism. When the Mughal Empire collapsed in the mid-1850s, the British took control of India.

Over centuries, Islam and Christianity were both imported into India. One of the results of the colonization is that Christianity is India's third-largest religion, after Hinduism and Islam, with nearly twenty-seven million followers, or a little over 2 percent of India's population, as per 2011 census data.

India is also home to the third-largest Muslim population, with around two hundred million Muslims, accounting for over 10 percent of the world's Muslim population. Hindus constitute 80 percent of the nearly 1.3 billion people who live in India.

Everyone in India has a lineage from other worlds. Much like the union of states that came together to make America, India was conceived as a union of five hundred princely states. It has twenty-two official languages, spoken across twenty-eight states and eight union territories that form the Republic of India.

Each state worships different deities, eats different cuisine, speaks different dialects, wears different clothes, and increasingly, as inequality has grown, does not get along with its neighbors.

Mumbai, modern India's financial engine, is the part of India where you find every other part of India.

The city is a collection of tropical islands framed by the Arabian Sea, making it exotic, overwhelming, spectacular, and cloyingly humid—like the India of storybooks. Over time, a megacity sprang around ruins of the empire, corroding artfully in the Indian summer.

Mumbai is a city where the old coexists with the even older. It's a city where everybody is from somewhere else and the absurd walks hand in hand with the mundane.

In conversations about the city, the residents will frequently compare it to the "other"—Delhi—with which Mumbai has a long-standing rivalry. Mumbai, its residents would tell you, wins because it has Bollywood—the world's largest film industry. And the city is every bit the blinged-out fantasy Bollywood makes it out to be. There are neighborhoods with glitzy salons and swanky restaurants overrun by celebrities. This is where Bollywood meets India Inc., the corporate leaders of modern India.

When fame meets power, there is an indecent amount of wealth on display.

When Mukesh Ambani, India's wealthiest man, got his daughter married in December 2018, Indian newspapers estimated the wedding cost at tens of millions of dollars. An appearance by Beyoncé is rumored to have cost the Ambani family $10 million.[1] Ambani gifted his daughter a fifty-thousand-square-foot multimillion-dollar mansion with sweeping views of the Arabian Sea.[2] The mansion is a short and luxurious drive to the Queen's Necklace, the promenade running alongside the sea. If viewed at night, the streetlights resemble a necklace of pearls. This Mumbai is clean, rich, and kinder to its residents and has remained the quintessential melting pot as history unfolded around it through wars and plagues and invaders and refugees.

The minute you zoom in, look beyond the stories of the quintessential melting pot, and gaze into the city's sprawling ghettos, Mumbai grabs you by the throat.

This Mumbai is poor, filthy, and unkind.

Neighborhoods are a sum total of the people who live there, and they, like people, have unique traits. They are welcoming or forbidding. Safe or hostile. Healthy or frail. The ghettos of Mumbai are so full of misery and injustice that they might as well be a planet away from the richer neighborhoods. They are filled with the poverty of lice and filth and wretched housing, infectious diseases and families sleeping twelve to one.

Not knowing about it is like knowing nothing of Mumbai itself.

There is as much concentrated poverty as there is concentrated wealth in Mumbai. For new visitors, there is enough of "rich Mumbai" to easily spend a lifetime without wandering into the belly of the beast—Mumbai, East Ward.

On the southeastern edges of Mumbai, not far from the shoreline of the Arabian Sea, looms a cluster of densely packed highrises, all measuring some 250 meters across at their widest. It is called the Natwar Parekh Compound, or NP Compound. Straight, cemented lanes cut across the complex of fifty-nine buildings, all seven stories tall and stacked only three meters apart.

These are Mumbai's vertical slums, the Indian equivalent of the Chicago Housing Authority's high-rise projects.

Roughly seventy thousand people make their homes in the NP Compound's forty-eight hundred matchbox-sized single-room living units.[3] It is the kind of high-density government housing that is unwelcoming and claustrophobic. The neighborhood serves as a visual reminder of many of Mumbai's greatest challenges: the desperate shortage of real estate, a growing population crisis, and a brewing public health nightmare that lurks in poorly designed urban housing. These buildings, a result of decades of residential segregation, perpetuate poverty, neglect, and health deficits among residents that is eerily similar to what happened in African American neighborhoods in the United States.

The density of construction warps perspective—when you look up from the narrow lanes, the buildings seem to stretch impossibly high. The sun does not reach the lower floors, so they remain in perpetual darkness, which has a perverse advantage: the poor families who work in shifts can sleep in shifts.

Even when it is not raining, it is best to venture inside NP Compound under an umbrella. Residents on the higher floors have a tendency to throw garbage and wastewater out of the windows. The monsoon season is hot, and the humid, thick air adds to the designed claustrophobia of the compound.

It makes the place smell different.

The neighborhood captures what is, for most Indians, an essence of poverty: the stench of rotting food and piles of garbage spoiling rapidly in the warm summer sun. Our response to strong, putrefying smells explains why we believed in the miasmatic theory for so many centuries. In places like the NP Compound, it is as if you can *feel* the disease in the air.

Few places in Mumbai are more hostile to life than its sprawling ghettos.

In July 2018, a small team of doctors working for a medical aid group called Doctors for You (DFY) made a startling announcement: the buildings constructed by Mumbai's state government were incubators of a tuberculosis epidemic.

The doctors had set up shop deep inside NP Compound, and much of their work focused on the Mumbai East Ward, where over 70 percent of residents live in slums. Mumbai East also has the world's densest concentration of people with drug-resistant tuberculosis, a nastier version of TB that is increasingly difficult to cure, as the bacteria has become resistant to even the most powerful antibiotics.

When DFY first moved into NP Compound in 2010, it combined three living units to create enough working space for a team of ten. The organization was originally set up as a health center, recognized by the state government to provide basic services such as vaccination and interventions in maternal and child health. Dr. Ravikant Singh, DFY's founder, recalled that the organization "immediately started seeing more and more TB patients, and got permission to start a DOTS centre"—where tuberculosis patients come for their daily course of directly observed treatment, the standard WHO-approved therapy against the disease.

"From there, it sort of snowballed," Dr. Singh told me when I interviewed him in August 2018.

By 2017, despite seven years of work, DFY's doctors had not seen any reduction in TB cases within these vertical slums. They realized that no matter how methodical they were in their anti-TB work, nothing made a difference. Their own data proved it: "We maintained detailed DOTS registers with information about where patients lived," said Dr. Peehu Pardeshi, an expert on the molecular biology of the tuberculosis bacterium.[4]

From those registers, "we had a hunch that something strange was afoot here."

Despite lack of funds and staff and the overwhelming needs of the community, doctors at DFY undertook a methodical deduction process that would have made Arthur Conan Doyle proud.

In July 2018, after a few days of thinking out loud, Dr. Singh, Peehu's boss and DFY's founder, had an idea: "I asked my DOTS staff to do a mapping of patients, building-wise." They pulled out an aerial shot of the fifty-nine buildings, checked the register, and started marking in red, next to each building, each patient living in it. When they were done, "there was a collective gasp," he recalled.

That aerial shot of the slum clusters is now known as the "trigger photo" within DFY. It was the first time DFY staff could visualize the scale of the health crisis. The photograph resembles a densely stacked honeycomb. There are fifty-nine rooftops, tiny squares, and red arrows coming out of them. Against each arrow, DFY researchers have put a number—to reflect how many TB patients live in each building. The markings get denser, more clustered, on the lower floors.

One building in particular stands out—building number 10 of the NP Compound. Researchers had found fifty-one drug-resistant (DR) TB patients in *one* building in one of Mumbai's sprawling ghettos—an exceptional find, even for a country like India. It was the equivalent of finding fifty-one people suffering from a rare cancer, all neighbors. At least one member of every family living inside building number 10 had DR TB. Not regular, curable, drug-sensitive TB, but the kind where the bacteria stop responding to antibiotics.

Over the next few days, Peehu Pardeshi approached the civil engineering department at the Indian Institute of Technology, Bombay, her alma mater. She wanted to know if the buildings themselves could be causing tuberculosis.

The "trigger photo" inspired a research project where doctors, architects, and government officials came together in ways that make one believe in the concept of good governance.[5] The report is a Kafkaesque bill of indictment, providing unimpeachable evidence that the slum redevelopment projects are a colossal failure and confirming them as one of the hottest of hotspots for DR TB in Mumbai, in India, and most likely in the world. The DFY researchers were alarmed but could not explain why exactly: "All families living in these buildings are of the same socioeconomic class. They earn the same amount, lived pretty much the same way. We couldn't understand why some of them were getting TB, and some were not," said Dr. Pardeshi.

In December 2008, the Slum Rehabilitation Authority, or SRA, was sold to Mumbai residents as the city's flagship achievement in "slum redevelopment"—to raze unauthorized slum clusters and move their residents into new, improved housing.

It would finally solve Mumbai's housing crisis, so people were told.

The government promised free housing to all slum dwellers who were in Mumbai prior to 1995, which effectively meant having to provide about eight million free homes.[6] Many of the high-rise colonies in the Mumbai East Ward, like NP Compound, were built as part of "redevelopment" efforts to make space for Mumbai's swelling population on the cleared slum land. Within a decade, three projects—all crown jewels of the Maharashtra government's SRA initiative—had become a petri dish of DR TB.[7] The projects were social engineering on a scale never seen before.

Decades later, India's TB outbreak is the biggest unintended consequence of a policy of residential segregation that turned houses into efficient incubators for the bacteria.[8] The TB outbreak in Mumbai, and across India, is the evil sum of India's deficiencies. The urban, vertical slums are where policy meets people. The SRA projects, much like projects in the US, are an indictment of the uneven distribution of prosperity in postindependence India. When I first visited this place, in August 2018, the structures made me think the words "concentration camps" and "panopticon" must have been on the architect's mind. They are singularly hideous and could only have been imagined by an architect on a government contract who designed, effectively, a cautionary tale for future city planners.

The first lesson is to never stack tall buildings so close together. It was done to save the Maharashtra government as much land as possible. The saved land was then sold at market value to private builders.

To the residents of rich Mumbai, the new densely packed buildings were the "solution" to a housing crisis that was a century in the making. What was framed as a solution was actually a problem arising from the cumulative effect of class and caste warfare, launched against the poorest and most vulnerable citizens of India.

Health deficits among India's poor, especially lower-caste communities, are parallel to health deficits in racially segregated neighborhoods in America. These are different names for the same system of oppression.

The housing crisis may have laid the groundwork for India's TB epidemic, but it is a far deeper social failing that *caused* the housing crisis.

* * *

Tuberculosis is a patient killer. Because TB patients don't die soon after being infected, they remain a reservoir of microbes, capable of spreading the deadly infection to their neighbors and colleagues every time they sneeze, cough, or spit in public.

TB thrives in dense populations, the kind that formed in the wake of the industrial revolution. From the bacteria's point of view, many human advancements have opened new opportunities to thrive. Railway systems allowed disease to spread faster than ever before. When transcontinental flights became common, infectious diseases like drug-resistant tuberculosis, once considered limited to faraway lands, became global. But the wider travels of populations do not, on their own, explain the rise in TB.

The bacteria thrived on one particular human folly: prejudice.

Industrialization led to a stampede of workers looking for employment moving from rural areas to urban areas. Upon reaching the cities, workers found that wretched and inadequate housing awaited them.

Mumbai's current outbreak is directly linked to TB's parallel journey with capital. Plagues are fueled by a deliberate architecture of unfairness. In Mumbai's case, profits from the British Empire, which financed the industrial revolution, came back to Mumbai in a metastasized manner, choking the tropical island with subhuman and unsafe housing.

The impact of industrialization on TB's spread was swift.

A 2015 paper on TB during the industrial revolution noted that "roughly 15% of all deaths in London before 1730 were due to the disease, a percentage that nearly doubled in the early 1800s."[9] The industrial revolution was exported to the colonized world under the banner of imperialism, and as in Europe and America, it led to overcrowding and, predictably, upward trends in TB incidence. The British East India Company transformed Bombay (as Mumbai was then known) into an urban center in the nineteenth century. By the middle of the century, Indian businessmen had set up textile mills to manufacture cotton for the empire. Bombay, which emerged to maintain a steady supply of cotton and opium, would soon pay a heavy price for its rapid urbanization.

Tuberculosis was not the only pathogen thriving in the fast-industrializing world in which diseases, and not wars, were the biggest killers. Bombay was shaped by one of the worst plagues in human history: the bubonic plague of 1896.

On September 23, 1896, the first case of bubonic plague was detected in Mandvi, a congested locality along the shore.[10] The island city's population at the time numbered over eight million, most of them immigrants who came to the city looking for jobs. The plague rapidly spread to all parts of the city, and the death toll was estimated at nineteen hundred people per week through the rest of the year.[11] This triggered panic among colonial officials, the commercial elite, and especially the businessmen who owned textile mills and needed labor. The rich fled the city.

A headline in the *New York Times* captured the disaster: "Fleeing from Bombay, Deserting the City to Escape the Bubonic Plague: More Than Half the Population Has Run Away, and Business Is Paralyzed—Cemeteries Filled with the Dead." Predictably, the brunt of the plague was borne by the poor, with mill workers emerging as the most exploited community. Even with eight million people, a fraction of its current population, Bombay's terrible housing conditions facilitated the spread of the disease. Initially, municipal officials sought to wish away the problem, but as the plague refused to subside and the death toll rose, commerce was affected. Relief operations were hesitantly started.

Without including Indians in the decision, the British colonizers thought that segregation and forced hospitalization were the most effective ways to contain the spread of the plague. A government order, passed on October 6, 1896, required all persons suspected of having the plague to be separated from the rest of the population. In 1897, the Epidemic Diseases Act was passed, which gave additional powers to the civic authorities to detain and isolate plague suspects and to inspect, disinfect, evacuate, and even demolish dwellings suspected of being contaminated. Fairs and pilgrimages were stopped, road and rail travelers detained for inspection.

British officials took measures that Indians found intrusive, violating the caste and community precepts of Indian society.[12] By late 1897, Bombay was facing an acute shortage of "cooks, tailors, barbers, coolies and mill workers." Colonial authorities feared a complete breakdown if municipal workers such as scavengers, sweepers, and drivers of municipal vans—significantly from lower-caste communities—joined the general exodus of persons fleeing the city. Officials realized that the plague would spiral out of control if they did not have people to clean the sewers, move the sick to hospitals, or carry the dead to the graveyards.[13] Railway and port authorities were ordered to refuse them tickets and, if necessary, detain them by force.

During the plague years, colonial authorities, as well as Bombay's rich traders, recognized the connection between disease transmission and overcrowding. Two years after the plague began, on November 9, 1898, the colonial state created the Bombay City Improvement Trust (BIT) through an Act of Parliament. The Municipal Corporation and the government handed over all vacant lands to this body—with the mandate to improve the city.

The BIT is one of the biggest failures in urban planning anywhere in the world. Everything that is wrong with Bombay's housing policy flows from the attempt by this authority to reconcile the need to keep poor people around to do menial work while separating them from the rich.

The promise of India's economic boom would remain physically separated from the poor, locked inside guarded gates and gated communities. Decisions made a century ago would inevitably lead us to the fragmented archipelago of enclaves that exist today, replacing previously integrated cities and communities.

The BIT, despite being created to improve housing conditions for the city's poorest classes, made it worse. The failure is captured in a paper titled "The Bombay Improvement Trust, Bombay Mill-owners and the Debate over Housing Bombay's Millworkers." It was written by Caroline E. Arnold, from the Department of Political Science at the University of New York.

Although both Bombay's commercial elite and millowners feared the disruption to the city's economic activities caused by the plague, neither the Improvement Trust nor the mills provided a long term solution to the problem of housing for Bombay's millworkers.

As of 1920, the Trust had constructed 21,387 tenements; it had also demolished 24,428.[14]

The body acted as a "slum clearance" board—making the slums disappear without solving the interlocked crisis of housing, health care, and employment. The trader castes—the mill owners—did not care about the housing crisis until it became impossible to hire workers.

Meanwhile, the BIT actively aggravated the housing crisis by demolishing and reducing the amount of available housing and, by doing so, raising the cost of what remained.

"Mill housing"—a precursor to the modern Bombay slums—was a direct response to difficulties in securing workers during the plague years. Employers had to offer acceptable housing to get labor. By the 1920s, seventeen of Bombay's eighty-six mills provided housing for some of their workers. N. N. Wadia, who ran Sir Dinshaw Petit's mills, constructed *chawls*—similar to tenements in New York City—to house at least twenty-five hundred (25 percent) of their ten thousand workers and their dependents. However, the majority of mill owners remained skeptical of providing housing, asserting that workers refused to live in chawls because "when they absented themselves from the mill, the jobber knew exactly where to find them."

The failure to provide large-scale housing was part of a broader failure of mill workers to organize on the "labor question"— whether in terms of wages, hours of work, or strikes. "Although a coordinated wage policy would have helped to reduce workers' movement across mills, such efforts would have similarly undercut each mill's ability to poach workers, attract workers with higher wages after the plague and strikes, and would have required citywide agreement on the level at which mills wages should be set," Arnold argued.[15]

To the benefit of mill owners, there was no standardization of wages, housing, or working hours. The BIT's failure was such that by 1920, even with the addition of BIT and private chawls to the city's housing stock, there was still a net deficit of housing for seventeen thousand individuals.

The few who did build chawls built them as dense, crowded clusters—all too familiar to anyone who has visited the city.

Between 1880 and 1940, there were no fewer than ten governmental investigations into labor conditions in India, which included Bombay's mills. The debates, typical of both Indian and British administrations, devolved into squabbling factions, each refusing to accept responsibility for the failure to build housing for the working classes.

Ultimately what passed as a "solution" for the housing crisis—it was nothing close—would eventually serve as a blueprint for residential segregation in Bombay, along both class and caste lines.

If the BIT's failure is chalked up to the colonial state's callousness, everything since independence has been a collective failure in urban planning by successive governments.

The city's ghettos would be for the workers, while the rich went the only way they could—upward—and built skyscrapers. In the 1950s and 1960s, the Maharashtra state government's initial response to overcrowding, learning no lessons from the BIT's failure, was slum clearance. Legally speaking, slums in India are unauthorized structures where the inhabitants do not have title to the land they occupy. The city bulldozed the huts and rehoused slum dwellers in subsidized rental housing. Once again, the approach did not work due to obvious lack of space. Once they realized that, the government took a more tolerant approach.

The new policy was "slum upgradation."

Under it, the government transferred the leasehold tenure of land to cooperative housing societies of slum dwellers. It also provided basic services such as water, toilets, electricity, streetlights, and primary health care and education to slum dwellers.

While better than the slum clearance policy, the scale of this program remained limited and did not prevent slum proliferation, which worsened when migrants flooded to the city in search of opportunities, hoping to find small corners in the big city.[16] The city cradled innovation and entrepreneurship and, consequently, saw urbanization at a dizzying, unprecedented scale in the twenty-first century.

The second phase of Mumbai's transformation was kickstarted in the 1990s with the economic liberalization of India. The country integrated with the global economy, leading to a rapid expansion of the upper class and a new middle class. There was proportionately rapid expansion of slums in urban centers, filled with lower-caste communities to serve the rapidly rising classes. The haves and the have-nots, crammed together tightly, learned to live cheek to jowl. The result was an explosion of walled islands and exclusionary collective spaces—a fragmented archipelago of enclaves such as gated communities, shopping malls, cineplexes, and office towers.

The megacity earned the epithet of Mayanagri—the city of dreams.

Lured by the happy-ending storylines of Bollywood's fantasies, migrants coming to Mumbai hoped their caste, gender, or background would not matter and that fortune would soon favor them. Living in Mumbai's slums became a part of the journey to becoming rich. That gave rise to another nickname for the city: Slumbai.

It was clear that both slum clearance and upgradation had failed. Most migrant families ended up permanently living on the margins, their dreams perpetually deferred. Mumbai was a city of outsiders looking in, hoping for a share in India's economic boom.

In 1995, the Maharashtra government came up with a new plan: this time, the strategy was slum redevelopment, out of which the SRA or Slum Rehabilitation Authority was born. With it, Mumbai became among the first cities in the world to adopt a free market solution to redevelop slum clusters.

Not surprisingly, it failed.

The new policies introduced various incentives for private developers in a bid to produce mass housing for the poor but without public spending. It meant that on plots occupied by slums, real estate developments were allowed to construct more buildings, closer together, with less open space than the normal regulations permitted. It also reduced the open space required on the side and rear of the buildings.

By 2011, Mumbai was home to 12.5 million people—with a population density of 19,600 people per square kilometer.[17] The rest of India, a famously crowded country, has a population density of 382 people per square kilometer. The Maharashtra government had, through its slum housing policies, picked super-dense housing—making communities living there a kind of petri dish for infectious diseases to thrive on. The government amended its land development law to make things much worse for the poor. A new set of regulations was added to deal exclusively with slum redevelopment schemes, basically institutionalizing antipoor building laws. Private developers were permitted to purchase slum land from the government at 25 percent of the market value—*if* they could obtain consent from 70 percent of the slum dwellers in the community.

The developers could, with the community's consent, clear the land and rehouse them. At the same time, builders were allowed—for the first time—to stack buildings just three meters apart instead of sixteen meters. So private developers offered slum dwellers the promise of new housing without explaining to them how densely packed the new boxes would be or how poor the plumbing would remain.

In December 2016, a workshop was organized at the Mumbai campus of the Tata Institute of Social Science to mark twenty years of slum redevelopment. The campus, also in Mumbai East, is a stone's throw from NP Compound, and social science students work closely with communities inside the vertical slums for research.

On the anniversary, numbers spoke louder than any story about the government's failures. Of the 1,524 redevelopment projects started, 197—or 13 percent—had been completed.[18] Just over 150,000 families had been "rehabilitated" over the two decades, against a promise of delivering eight hundred thousand units in the first five years of the policy.

No city in the world had segregated the rich from the poor, the lower caste from the upper castes, as efficiently as Mumbai. "The housing segregation didn't just happen by coincidence. It was a state-sponsored system of segregating people on income differences," added Dr. Singh, DFY's founder. While it maintained India's caste and class prejudices, the residential segregation reaped enormous rewards for private developers.

One of Mumbai's most prominent real estate projects, Imperial Towers, a twin-tower luxury residential skyscraper complex in South Mumbai, is built on former slum land. It is one of India's tallest buildings and one of the country's most expensive real estate projects with each condominium, of more than four thousand square feet, costing between US$3 million and US$5 million.[19] While the wealthy citizens built upward, there was no escaping the neighborhood below, which was a sprawl of corrugated iron–roofed huts below. It gave Mumbai the unique look of a city with "villages that had been airdropped into gaps between elegant modernities," wrote Pulitzer Prize–winning journalist Katherine Boo from her book, *Behind the Beautiful Forevers*.

Mumbai is a checkerboard of neighborhoods where the world's richest, with lifestyles similar to the high society in New York or London or Paris, live right next to entire neighborhoods whose lives are measured in human development indices. The first official population survey conducted by the government of Mumbai stated that about 8 percent of its population was living in slums in 1956. That number increased to 41.3 percent by 2011 and to 55 percent by 2018.[20] The Mumbai East Ward had the highest density of slums in the city, with 72.5 percent of the ward's population living in slums.

These slums were incubators of deadly drug-resistant bacteria.

As per the WHO, globally, an estimated 10 million people fell ill with TB in 2019.[21] An estimated 1.2 million died, India accounting for 31 percent of those deaths. Of the total infected, nearly 206,030 people were diagnosed with DR TB, a 10 percent increase from 186,883 in 2018.

The most DR TB patients, 66,255 to be precise, live in India.

The highest number of children infected with TB, 109,816, live in India. The highest number of health workers with TB also live in India. The WHO records 22,314 cases among health-care workers from seventy-six countries; India accounts for 47 percent and China for 18 percent.

Within India, the hotspot was, unsurprisingly, Maharashtra, with nearly 10,621 DR TB cases, 4,367 of them in Mumbai.[22] Globally, there are only 12,350 XDR, or extensively drug-resistant, TB cases in the world; two hundred of them live in Mumbai.[23]

The numbers reveal the interlocking crisis of poverty, poor immunity, and large family size—all exacerbated by the unintended outcome of the Maharashtra government's housing policy. Throughout medical history, the creation of concentrated pockets of infectious diseases has resulted in boomeranging circles of infections that inevitably ricochet outward, breaching all perceivable bubbles of race, caste, and class as they spread. More than any other type of disease, the spread of infectious diseases is dictated by human folly and prejudices.

As the mutated disease rises from the bowels of the inner city, it has become a rare truly democratizing factor in India, a nation with deep historic and congenital defects.

Now, seventy-five years after India's independence, the tuberculosis outbreak is a reckoning with a deeper flaw, and India's original sin: casteism.

* * *

"To the Untouchables," B. R. Ambedkar wrote in 1945, "Hinduism is a veritable chamber of horrors."

Ambedkar was a prophet from the future, a brilliant legal mind, and a complete wild card among the founding fathers of modern India. He stood at the rocking cradle of India's freedom movement and went on to become a leading jurist during her struggle for independence.

While Mohandas Karamchand Gandhi—better known by his honorific, Mahatma (Hindi word for a "great soul")—is the most recognizable of India's founding fathers, it is Bhimrao Ramji Ambedkar who was her fiercest social justice leader. While Gandhi, an upper-caste Hindu, focused on international threat, Ambedkar held the mirror to India's ruling class, which had subjugated oppressed castes for centuries.

No founding father grappled with misery at such a personal level as Ambedkar. He was born in 1891, into a Mahar family, lowest among India's castes, and faced discrimination as a result of it.

Lower castes were formerly known as "Untouchables" in India. *Dalit* is the Marathi word for "broken but resilient people," and it has been in use since the 1880s as a term of self-determination and self-identification of lower-caste communities.[24]

Ambedkar's father served in the British Indian Army stationed in the Central Provinces (now Madhya Pradesh), making him a rare lower-caste child to attend school. Even though his family had the means to educate him, he and his friends were not allowed to sit inside the class along with upper-caste students. Teachers would not touch his notebooks, and "Untouchable" students could not drink water from the taps "touchable" upper-caste students used. If the peon, an unskilled helper hired by the school, did not assist them, Dalit students would go thirsty all day.

"While in the school I knew that children of the touchable classes, when they felt thirsty, could go out to the water tap, open it, and quench their thirst.... But my position was separate. I could not touch the tap; and unless it was opened for me by a touchable person, it was not possible for me to quench my thirst," Ambedkar wrote in 1936.

After graduating from high school, Ambedkar studied economics and political science at Elphinstone College in Bombay University, where he met Sayajirao Gaekwad III, the maharaja of the princely state of Baroda. The maharaja, an active advocate of social reforms, including the removal of untouchability, sponsored Ambedkar's higher education, first at Columbia University in New York, where he completed a masters and a PhD, and later at the London School of Economics.

In 1917, as Europe inched closer to war, he came back to India to be rudely reminded of this "untouchability." From London, he went to Baroda, honor bound. "Since I had been educated by the Baroda State, I was bound to serve the State," he later wrote in his personal entries.[25] At Baroda Station, faced with the question of finding lodging, Dr. Ambedkar froze. "My five years of staying in Europe and America had completely wiped out of my mind any consciousness that I was an untouchable, and that an untouchable wherever he went in India was a problem to himself and to others."

Hindu hotels wouldn't take him, and he was not keen on impersonating a Hindu to get lodging. He eventually decided to go to a Parsi inn (Parsis follow the Zoroastrian religion, which does not recognize untouchability). Soon after his check-in, the Parsi innkeeper questioned Ambedkar's identity. "Not knowing that this inn was maintained by the Parsi community for the use of Parsis only, I told him that I was a Hindu."

The innkeeper, in need of money, hosted him but registered him under a Parsi name. Ambedkar managed to stay at this inn, in a storage space in the attic, for eleven days before being found out and confronted by a dozen angry-looking Parsis. They accused him of "polluting" the Parsi inn and asked him to leave the inn that very day. He told a coworker, a Hindu, about his housing crisis; the coworker was indignant and sad but did not offer to help.

In his diaries, Ambedkar recounted the Hindu friend saying, "If you come to my home, my servants will go." Ambedkar spent the next five hours at a public garden in Kamathi Baug and left for Bombay by the night train.

A century later, Dalit communities face similar struggles in finding housing.

By 1918, he was teaching political economics at the Sydenham College of Commerce and Economics at Bombay University. He still could not drink from the common tap. This time it was faculty members, his colleagues, who refused to share it with him.

When India became independent in August 1947, Prime Minister Jawarharlal Nehru invited Ambedkar to be the first minister of law and justice. Shortly after, the Constituent Assembly appointed him chair of the drafting committee for the new constitution. This would be his defining legacy.

He was the right person, in the right place, at the right time—his will equal parts velvet and iron. The profits from his struggles were India's.

After two years of town halls, amendments, and negotiations, on January 24, 1950, the final draft of the Indian constitution was ready—in two languages, Hindi and English.

The document had 395 articles at the time of drafting, in twenty-two parts and twelve schedules from cover to cover. It is thirty times larger than the US Constitution by size and has been amended 104 times, compared to twenty-seven amendments to the US Constitution. Ambedkar was particularly influenced by equality legislation in the US Constitution and said he had "borrowed from the [American] Civil Rights Protection Acts, 1866," the results of which are enshrined in Articles 14 (equal protection under law), 15, 16 (anti discrimination laws), and 17 (abolishment of untouchability) of the Indian Constitution.[26]

In 1946, Ambedkar contacted W. E. B. Du Bois to inquire about the National Negro Congress petition to the UN, which attempted to secure minority rights through the UN. "As a student at Columbia, Dr. B. R. Ambedkar studied with some of the greatest figures of interwar American liberalism, such as John Dewey and Edward Seligman, and American historians James Shotwell and James Harvey Robinson. Dewey, an American philosopher and educational reformer, was Dr. Ambedkar's intellectual mentor at Columbia University."[27]

He told Du Bois that he had been a "student of the Negro problem" and that "there is so much similarity between the position of the Untouchables in India and of the position of the

Negroes in America that the study of the latter is not only natural but necessary."[28]

On July 31, 1946, Du Bois responded by saying he would send Ambedkar a copy and that he had "every sympathy with the Untouchables of India."[29] Not coincidentally, the caste equality movement in India has continued to draw inspiration from the American civil rights movement. The Dalit Panthers were established in 1972, directly inspired by the Black Panthers in the US.

Ambedkar had hammered into the constitution provisions and safeguards for minorities, alongside the emphatic abolition of untouchability. His vision of a generous, inclusive India has driven the country for seventy-five years. He believed the innate structural inequality of Indian society could only be fixed with the "annihilation" of caste.

He was also a pioneering feminist and the reason why Indian women had the right to vote at the time of the nation's birth. He aimed his ax as much at misogyny as he did at casteism. He argued that control of women's bodies through child marriage and restriction of widow remarriage were all devised to deal with the problem of "surplus women" while keeping the caste groups enclosed.

The constitution is not a perfect document by any means, but it was a significant moment of progress in the history of newly independent India.

Speaking after the completion of his work, Ambedkar said, "I feel that the Constitution is workable; it is flexible and it is strong enough to hold the country together both in peace time and in war time. Indeed, if I may say so, if things go wrong under the new Constitution the reason will not be that we had a bad Constitution. What we will have to say is that Man was vile."[30]

And man was vile.

The promise of India did not extend to the lower caste and class, who she still holds in forced exile from her triumphs. Even though "untouchability" was formally abolished in 1950, seventy-five years of independence have not been enough to erase this two-thousand-year-old social hierarchy. Under this system, Hindu society is categorized, divided into rigid hierarchical groups based on their karma, deeds, and dharma, an elastic framework laying down duties, rights, laws, conduct, virtues, and "right way of living" as per Hindu scripture.

Caste, to this day, defines a person's place in society, what jobs they can do, who they can marry, and if they can share water from the same drinking source. The top three castes—priests, warriors, and traders—are upper castes.

The fourth, Shudra, are lower castes but still within the Brahminic caste system. The fifth, Dalits, are considered so lowly that they are outside the caste system; they are outcasts. Their place in the social order is to do menial jobs: cleaning toilets, sweeping streets, burning dead bodies, and so forth.

The word "Dalit" was popularized by Ambedkar. The term now also serves as a political identity, similar to how the LGBTQ community reclaimed "queer" from its pejorative use and turned it into a positive self-identifier and a political identity. Millions of people, about 17 percent of India's population of 1.3 billion, continue to be treated as Untouchable by their fellow citizens.

While contemporary horrors like apartheid in South Africa and the Jim Crow era in America have been internationally challenged, India's practice of caste, an insidious and brutal system of hierarchy, has managed to escape similar scrutiny and censure.

Writer Arundhati Roy argues that this is "perhaps because it has come to be so fused with Hinduism, and by extension with so much that is seen to be kind and good—mysticism, spiritualism, non-violence, tolerance, vegetarianism, Gandhi, yoga, backpackers, the Beatles—that, at least to outsiders, it seems impossible to pry it loose and try to understand it."

Making matters worse, caste is not visible. It is not color-coded.

With rapid urbanization, and the ghettos that came with it, India's lower castes were forced into social isolation. For centuries, Dalit communities have been forced to work as cleaners, manual scavengers, street cleaners, and waste pickers, causing health deficits that are mirrored in low-income communities around the world. Like poorer communities in the US or UK, families living on the margins of India's society did not have reliable access to education, health care, or legal aid.

The colonial period concretized this social order by distributing land titles and land ownership to upper-caste Indians. A study from 2018, titled "Wealth Inequality, Class and Caste in India, 1961–2012," provided data to enumerate what has always been true about India: that caste plays a significant role in the educational and professional choices available to citizens and directly impacts income and assets.

A separate report called "Wealth Ownership and Inequality in India: A Socio-Religious Analysis," conducted jointly by three universities, found that 22.3 percent of the country's upper-caste Hindus owned 41 percent of the country's total wealth, forming the richest group in India.[31]

The households in the top 1 percent (in terms of wealth) owned 25 percent of the country's total assets, while the top 5 percent owned 46 percent of it. In stark contrast, the bottom 40 percent of households were found to own just 3.4 percent of the country's total assets.

This is not too different from the growing racial wealth gap in the US.

According to the 2019 Federal Reserve data, the top 1 percent of Americans have a combined net worth of $34.2 trillion (or 30.4 percent of all household wealth in the US), while the bottom 50 percent of the population holds just $2.1 trillion combined (or 1.9 percent of all wealth).[32]

In India, the richest state was Maharashtra, and the highest valued asset—as in colonial times—was land. Nowhere is land more precious than Maharashtra's capital city, Mumbai. Mumbai's neighborhoods are segregated along caste, class, and religion such that it has become the textbook definition of the ghettoization of minorities.

This rigid social order spills over generation after generation.

In Mumbai's poorest neighborhoods, life expectancy is as unpredictable, brutal, and by extension, short as it was a century ago. While residential segregation in US and Europe have been extensively studied, India has not yet done that. We know from US and European experience that residential segregation aggravates existing socioeconomic inequality.

In 2019, researchers at Cornell University presented the first ever neighborhood-scale study of segregation patterns in India's major urban centers—Delhi, Mumbai, Bengaluru, Chennai, and Kolkata. The paper, titled "Isolated by Caste: Neighbourhood-Scale Residential Segregation in Indian Metros," argued that the practice of residential segregation increased the concentration of poverty among the minorities in India exactly the same way as it did in the US, drawing parallels with the socioeconomic conditions prior to one of the worst riots in recent American history—the Los Angeles riots of 1992.

The riots were the result of many underlying social conditions—racism, social injustice, and poverty. The living conditions in South Central Los Angeles in the years prior to the riots were below average. The per capita income was less than half that of Los Angeles as a whole, and poverty and unemployment rates were more than twice as high. Additionally, drugs, crime, and gang violence had all become visible problems.

The authors made a comparison to note that the "Los Angeles riots of 1992, for example, was due to highly segregated residential neighborhoods with 'unequal social and political endowments and economic niches.'"[33]

Segregation of residential areas on caste/race lines results, inevitably, in concentration of poverty. In Indian cities, individuals are routinely denied access to housing of their choice based on their caste identity.

In 1971, American economist Thomas Schelling wrote a seminal paper called "Models of Segregation," revealing how inadvertent choices—like the simple act of denial or a small preference for one's neighbors to be of the same caste/race—could lead to total segregation.[34] A direct impact of this segregation is on the distribution of public services and goods that come to define neighborhoods as "good" and "bad." Bad neighborhoods, where supposedly no one is innocent and everyone deserves whatever befalls them, are characterized by poor municipal services like garbage collection, sewage treatment, hospitals, and schools—all of which is used to further dehumanize the poor.

Around the world, the ghettoes of megacities like Mumbai are described with words such as "dirty" and "dangerous," and these can be used to describe the people who live there as well as the neighborhood itself.

This medical dystopia is more than the sum of its squalid parts, says Dr. Singh, who has now spent a decade working in Mumbai's ghettoes. "People routinely blame residents of these colonies for it being filthy. That the chawls are decrepit is further used as an argument to reinforce discrimination. As if the ghetto were a ghetto because of the people who lived there, and not because the government failed them. It is also common to use the poverty and decrepitude of chawls to cast aspersions on the character and habits of the residents—there is too much crime here."

The tool that gives social sanction for this condemnation is caste.

The TB outbreak in Mumbai, and across India, is the evil sum of India's deficiencies. Patients routinely die from TB in the county. But what kills them? It is everything, including their airless, humid rooms; the single toilet shared by at least fifty people; and a lack of information, resources, and, most of all, empathy.

Poverty is the disease, TB the symptom.

The global fight against TB will be won, or more likely lost, in India because a century of bad housing policy decisions has meant that Mumbai's rich residents live in their gated luxury archipelago of enclaves high in the sky while keeping the poor residents of Mumbai in serving distance as their cooks and drivers and security guards and lift operators.

Together, but separated more than ever. For the bacteria, this is a great opportunity to thrive.

In 2000, Amitabh Bachchan, Bollywood superstar and Mumbai's most famous resident, was diagnosed with TB in the spine. The diagnosis came right before the launch of the first edition of the TV show *Kaun Banega Crorepati*, the Indian version of *Who Wants to Be a Millionaire*.

Wealth or caste cannot protect anyone from the miseries that are inflicted upon the inner cities. Tuberculosis is no longer a disease only of the poor or an abstract threat from history.

In India, where the rich and the poor live less than a sneeze away, their destinies hopelessly intermingled, it is the daily business of life.

* * *

If the TB bacteria can withstand two antibiotic drugs, it is known as multidrug-resistant tuberculosis, or MDR TB.[35] If it can resist four drugs, it is called extensively drug-resistant tuberculosis, or XDR TB. The chemotherapy for DR TB is far more dangerous than treatment for drug-sensitive TB, the kind in which the bacteria is still sensitive to antibiotics.

Treatment for DR TB can last up to two years, whereas for regular, drug-sensitive TB, treatment is a six-month therapy. The Western world has seen a slow decline in TB, thanks to housing reform, slum clearance, and new medical interventions that came with increasing prosperity. Once the Western world found TB to be curable, the research and funding into new treatments dried up. Meanwhile, in parts of the world that did not gain from industrialization to the same degree that Western economies did, the crisis was snowballing.

The WHO, cognizant of the growing threat, introduced DOTS—the international protocol for treating TB—in 1994. The most striking feature of the DOTS strategy was the amount of distrust it showed toward TB patients. Within the global health community, the DOTS strategy is now considered to have failed, with the main evidence for this failure being the rise of drug-resistant TB around the world.

Unlike any other disease where patients are given their medicines and expected to follow the doctor's advice, the DOTS strategy expected TB patients to turn up at a DOTS clinic every day at the same time for six months so a health worker could watch the patient swallow their pills. Many employers fire TB patients for being routinely late to or absent from work just because they are taking their medicine on time.

Unsurprisingly, most patients stop coming for treatment because of the physical challenge of swallowing eight to twenty pills at once for months. It is not just the number of pills; the toxicity of this treatment makes it just as bad as chemotherapy for cancer patients. The old-generation drugs, still being used to treat TB, are terrible to ingest, they burn the insides, patients sometimes lose taste, and they have crippling side effects, including deafness, weight loss, and suicidal depression.

The DOTS center in NP Compound is the size of a regular unit in the building. It has 225 square feet and is one-third the size of DFY's office, which is situated one floor above. The clinic is sparsely furnished, with a few plastic chairs, two floor fans, a few cupboards to store drugs, and medical files. On the wall facing the entrance, the staff has listed annual TB cases in the neighborhood since 2011. There are more charts of TB data, and on a whiteboard the doctors have the 2018 tally displayed:

- 29 DR TB patients under treatment in August 2017
- 22 of them have TB in the lungs, pulmonary TB
- 7 cases extra-pulmonary—the kind involving organs other than the lungs (e.g., lymph nodes, bone marrow, spine, brain)

Over time the clinic started providing health services to residents in and around the ward who come for routine health checkups, immunization, family planning, dental, and ophthalmic services.

Tuberculosis prevention and control, however, has remained DFY's main priority. "The residents fall sick and come to us. So we know who has TB and who doesn't. But they don't want it known to their neighbors. They don't talk to each other about it," said Dr. Pardeshi in an interview at her office in August 2018.

The poverty of some patients is extreme, as are their medical needs.

When Dr. Pardeshi went to see where one new TB patient lived, on a follow-up visit, she found the patient's chawl contained nothing except a stove. "She came to the clinic *after* she had a miscarriage. She coughed so much that the fetus aborted," remembered Dr. Pardeshi, amazed that the patient had survived. The woman recovered but was soon pregnant again, which meant she was sick again, her immune system compromised by the demands of the pregnancy. The patient had no support from her family; her husband did not understand that she was in no position to become a mother; she had to go through the experience alone.

"There is so much stigma, they don't even tell their families or neighbors about it. Patients know they'll be ostracized—which is possible—even in a cramped space like this one," added Dr. Pardeshi.

When the area's DOTS worker, Shaheena Shaikh, arrives at 10:00 a.m., she finds patients already queuing up to get their daily dose of antibiotics. She opens the only window in the room, switches on the ceiling fan, then switches on a floor fan placed right behind her head. Controlling airflow in the room is important, as she will spend the rest of her day in a small room with tuberculosis patients prone to coughing bouts.

Over twelve to eighteen months, TB patients have to ingest 14,000–20,000 pills. This is the primary reason the DOTS strategy is "directly observed." The government appoints a person to watch you swallow the pills because most patients, with frail bodies and failing minds, cannot stay the course on their own.

When patients give up, the pathogen wins.

* * *

A consistent feature of India's TB epidemic has been the Indian government's steadfast denial of the scale of the problem.

In July 2018, after eight years of research, DFY shared the "trigger photo" and their research with the Maharashtra government. It was unimpeachable evidence that the housing design and segregation laid the groundwork for the TB outbreak they were witnessing. This was not a twist of fate but the inevitable outcome of a government policy and a state-sponsored system of residential segregation that had snowballed into a public health nightmare.

"When I first shared the trigger photo with M-East ward officials, they straight up told me—this was not possible. They were surprised. But we knew our data was thorough; there was no doubt in our mind. We matched our data with theirs. They denied till they could not deny it anymore," Dr. Singh told me over Skype in August 2018. "In the name of slum redevelopment, we have dumped poor people in Nazi ghetto-like colonies that are nightmarish to live in. The children of wealthy people in Mumbai need parks to play, schools to go to, and space for their cars. Look at this colony—the only recreational space here is a police station."

DFY researchers found evidence to corroborate two important things: First, there is a direct correlation between the height of the building and tuberculosis—families living on lower floors have more TB cases because they have less access to sunlight and fresh air. Second, the disease affects more women, and especially women of reproductive age, since they are most likely to be home-bound.[36] The researchers calculated sky-view factors, daylight factors, and air velocity and natural ventilation in the house and found that less than 20 percent of all indoor space was getting natural light. All fifty-nine buildings in the NP Compound face each other, and most windows aren't used, further causing short-age of fresh air and sunlight.

Residents on upper floors toss garbage out of their windows because of the lack of a functioning trash collection system, and since it can fall into the chawls below if the windows are left open, the residents there tend to shut them.

Even on the upper floors, residents are reluctant to use all their windows for ventilation—because in a house of 225 square feet, every inch is precious. When families buy a fridge or a cupboard, the window is often the only wall they can put it against.

The worst buildings are those in the middle of this cluster, which is where building number 10, with its fifty-one DR TB patients, is. In July 2018, Dr. Singh's organization submitted the damning eighty-one-page report, demanding that the apartheid building laws that allowed such terrible homes for the poor be scrapped. "Compactly stacked buildings are acting like culture medium/breeding ground for the TB bacteria," the DFY study concluded.[37]

"It is not enough to construct tall buildings. We have to make sure these buildings are conducive to the growth of people who live in them. If we don't address this, treating TB is pointless. We can go on pretending to treat patients, but we are not addressing basic issues causing this epidemic. We can forget eliminating TB by 2025. We won't even be able to control it in the next fifty years," Dr. Singh told me.

The report concluded bluntly, "In a bid to provide formal housing for maximum number of people on high value land, the DCRs have compromised on the basic standards for livability for the poor. Our planning norms are now aiding a public health disaster. . . . The city government must take necessary actions to bring improvements in housing and avert a public health crisis."[38]

The Maharashtra state government has since increased the distance between buildings in the new slum-redevelopment projects from the current three meters to six meters in newer chawls—still much less than the sixteen-meter distance that is mandatory for private buildings.

"What is built is built, we cannot change it now," Pardeshi said. But in the future, she continued, the report should be taken into consideration before constructing new rehabilitation projects. "In fact, you don't need this research to see that the design is bad—you only need eyes. There is a reason why private housing has strict rules."

DFY also submitted a proposal to the state government asking for an intensive campaign targeting tuberculosis. Most of Mumbai's TB patients don't wear masks, even though they are required to, to limit the spread of infection. In a tropical, overcrowded, humid place, it is not an easy request. Putting a face mask on adds to the stigma the patients face: neighbors find out, tongues wag, and before you know it, the family has no friends.

And in Mumbai's poor neighborhoods, life can be very hard without friends.

One of Dr. Pardeshi's patients with XDR TB was a twenty-four-year-old woman named Anita. Newly married, she had been sent back home by her in-laws after her diagnosis. (It is incorrectly believed that TB can cause women to be infertile, leading to divorces or abandonment by the husband, as was the case with Anita.) She was diagnosed with TB in her bones. Anita's family kept the diagnosis hidden from neighbors, so a visit from the doctor took them by surprise.

The family did most of the talking; Anita barely spoke to Dr. Pardeshi. Anita's mother told the doctor the TB caused her bones to hurt a lot, there was swelling in the joints, and her biggest challenge was to go down seven floors to the DOTS clinic to pick up her medicines. It took Anita an hour to climb down, stopping at each step, gritting her teeth against the pain. At the clinic she spent a few hours each day on the ground floor until she had gained the strength needed to make the climb back up.

As Dr. Pardeshi completed the checkup and took her leave, Anita unexpectedly spoke, telling the doctor to not worry about her. "It is not easy, but I can at least walk in and out of the building. The old never come down," she said quietly.

"Old people move in and only come back down as dead bodies."

CHAPTER 6

———◆———

ANTIBIOTIC APOCALYPSE,
ON THE MOVE

On May 7, 2018, Mohan Kumar checked into a hotel in Tokyo's business district.[1] He'd had an anxious flight from Mumbai, during which he had obsessively gone over the contents of the "big box file" he was carrying.

Mohan's eleven-year-old daughter, Piya, had been diagnosed with XDR TB in her ankle bone. Her life hinged on him getting entry into the building he was staring at. Mohan spent the night pacing around the bed, waiting for the sun to rise.

"My cousin knew some people in Tokyo. I asked him to help me meet someone, anyone, who worked in Otsuka." His voice trailed away. He was sure that if he could explain to them how badly his daughter needed delamanid, a drug created by the Japanese company, they'd understand.

Piya's treating physician, Dr. Zarir Udwadia, one of Mumbai's best chest physicians, had prescribed the drug and put him in touch with someone at the pharmaceutical company. Mohan hoped that would be enough to get him a face-to-face meeting.

A lawyer by training, he had made sure all the paperwork was perfectly prepared, the test results neatly arrayed, ordered by date. He had even indexed it. As soon as the company agreed to meet him, he took the first flight out of Mumbai. The following day, Mohan walked in at 3:00 p.m. sharp, and officials from Otsuka Pharmaceuticals accompanied him to a conference room. They had hired an interpreter.

Over the next hour, Mohan put up his exhibition of x-rays, postsurgery photos, medical files, and prescriptions that had consumed his life and his daughter's. He showed close-ups of his daughter's "debridement" surgeries—when a doctor scoops out the damaged tissue from a pus-filled wound—an excruciating process with a long recovery period.

Piya had gone through this surgery twice already. The lesions were causing her to walk with an uneven gait—it had been the symptom that had led to the diagnosis of TB. If the family did not get access to delamanid, she would have to go through the surgery every month. During her last debridement, Alia, her mother, had to restrain her screaming child as a doctor gouged into her wound.

Mohan had fainted.

The family was determined not to enter into this monthly nightmare. Mohan knew that he simply "had to get the drug." XDR TB is nothing like regular, drug-sensitive TB. The thousand-pill regime is ineffective against XDR TB. Only two drugs offer any hope. In 2018, delamanid, a new antibiotic, showed positive results in treating DR TB, particularly in children. Even though the drug was approved in 2014, it had not been registered in India. So Mohan had to fly to Japan to get it.

At the meeting, Otsuka's officials cross-questioned Mohan. He asked them questions too. The interrogation went on for an hour, and eventually the officials of Otsuka Pharmaceuticals informed Mohan that the meeting was over. They'd get back to him. Late that night, he woke up to his phone vibrating. It was an email notification from the company "saying my daughter's medicine is approved."

Piya was being given access to delamanid as a "compassionate use" case—a practice of providing drugs to patients for free on a case-by-case basis. This is the norm if the drugs are either expensive or yet to be approved by drug regulators.

On May 21, 2018, Mohan's fortieth birthday, Piya was put on delamanid—one of just 187 Indian patients to get access to it. For thousands of patients, unicorn tears were easier to come by.

"It is the greatest gift I have received," he said.

* * *

Zarir F. Udwadia is not just a good doctor; he is famously good. He is brilliant, kind, and expensive; he talks in a rapid-fire staccato.

He is the kind of doctor who has an army of people, medical staff, juniors, walking behind him on bedside rounds. People—students, families, juniors, and journalists—take notes when he talks. Every second of his day is carefully budgeted to benefit the most patients.

If you have TB, getting an appointment with Dr. Udwadia is like getting an audience with God. Your life depends on it, literally. And it takes a small miracle to get an appointment.

On March 31, 2019, at a small conference hall in Sofitel Hotel in Mumbai's Bandra Kurla Complex, Dr. Udwadia got up on the dais to speak about tuberculosis. He used his words efficiently, each one measured, spoken for a reason. Most of the people in the room knew enough about TB for him to dive right in—Hinduja

Hospital is one of Mumbai's prestigious privately run medical facilities.

He started his speech by telling the audience that tuberculosis in India was a play written by Anton Chekov and Franz Kafka—names chosen no doubt because both writers died of TB in their early forties. Over the next few minutes, he set the stage for a dystopian epic set in a shambolic world with one villain: the private sector doctor.

In India, this refers to doctors who are either self-employed and run small mom-and-pop neighborhood clinics or those who work in India's vast self-regulated and rather posh chain of private hospitals.

Dr. Udwadia was a rare voice in India's private sector—he had been taking on the fight from within the private medical profession, like a modern-day Semmelweis.

His attack on private sector doctors as the "villains" is based on a study published in 1991 that changed his career. He had just returned from London and started practicing at Hinduja Hospital when he read about a study conducted in Dharavi, Asia's largest slum settlement.

The findings were so disturbing they stayed with him.

The researchers had asked one fairly simple question to 105 private sector doctors: What regime do you prescribe to tuberculosis patients weighing 50 kilograms (110 pounds)?

With tuberculosis, as with many treatments, the correct dosage is influenced by a patient's weight. Only ten doctors—9.5 percent of the sample—correctly prescribed the drugs.[2] "There were eighty different types of prescriptions—most were inappropriate," Dr. Udwadia recounted to the audience in the conference hall.

A year later, in 1992, Dr. Udwadia diagnosed his first MDR TB patient, a teenage hemophiliac called Zubin Irani. He had

MDR before it became a public health buzzword. Irani set Dr. Udwadia off on a personal journey for the next two decades.

Dr. Udwadia recounts the experience as follows on his website:

In desperate attempts to cure him I wrote to the foremost UK TB expert at the time, Prof Peter Davies, who was generous with his advice. Zubin sadly died of his disease but Peter and I became friends, and he invited me to write the chapter on MDR-TB in India in his textbook, *Clinical Tuberculosis*.

Around this time I set up my free TB OPD at the Hinduja Hospital, where in the early years MDR was rare. It's been operating every Monday for the last 25 years, and is now the busiest clinic in the hospital.[3]

Over the two and a half decades, Dr. Udwadia has had a ringside seat to the relentless amplification of India's TB epidemic. This spiraling epidemic has progressed in perfect tandem with two neat parallels in India's health sector: underinvestment in public spending and unregulated growth of the private sector.

In the 1980s, the Indian government permitted the operation of bank-funded private hospitals in the country. As the population boomed, the government realized the crumbling hospitals it ran could not cater to patients, especially the rich, upper-class, upper-caste patients who expected bedside manners and dignity at hospitals.

Just as it had with land regulation, the Indian government looked for a free market solution.

Since the 1980s, the Indian government has relied on for-profit solutions to the country's growing health challenges. During that time the vast and self-regulated (which is to say, not at all regulated) private sector has midwifed the birth of India's TB epidemic.

To diagnose TB, doctors need to identify it first.

Dr. Udwadia was confident that most Indian doctors did not know how to diagnose or treat TB. Twenty-first-century Indian doctors, much like the nineteenth-century European doctors Semmelweis faced, do not like it when their competence is questioned. So, in 2010, Dr. Udwadia did a copycat study of the question asked in 1991. He conducted the same experiment in the same geographical area as the first one, Dharavi. It was still Asia's largest slum settlement.

This time, Dr. Udwadia added another question: What regime do you prescribe to a fifty-kilogram patient with MDR TB?

To Dr. Udwadia's horror, only 6 doctors of the 106 present gave the correct answer to the updated question. Instead, "there were about 63 different types of prescriptions"—most of which would serve as "only amplifying resistance. . . . Poor prescribing practice is a major factor fueling the MDR-TB epidemic," the study stated.[4] The rise in cases of DR TB in India is the ultimate result of using effective drugs ineffectively.

The study revealed the looming catastrophe created by poor data, bad governance, and an army of rogue private doctors. Most Indian private sector doctors were amplifying drug resistance instead of curing the disease, en masse.

"Allopaths seem willfully ignorant, to me. If the 1991 [study] predicted MDR, the 2011 study predicts the spread of the worst strains of DR TB," Dr. Udwadia told me in frustration.

Eight years later, a team led by Dr. Madhukar Pai, a TB specialist and director of McGill International TB Centre at McGill University in Montreal, conducted their own version of this study.

The team hired twenty-four actors, trained them to act like TB patients, and had them walk into clinics of private doctors in Mumbai and Patna. They presented with every key symptom: persistent cough for three weeks, fever, weight loss, night chills. The actors had over two thousand interactions with private doctors in Mumbai and Patna.[5]

Only 35 percent of 2,652 "cases" were diagnosed correctly.

In later versions of the study, the actor-patients even shouted, "I had TB in the past!" But some *still* failed to get a correct diagnosis. The doctors didn't believe them. Those who were diagnosed were then offered cocktails of inappropriate treatments ranging from broad-spectrum antibiotics and cough syrups to vitamins, homeopathy, and Ayurvedic (traditional healing) treatments.

Separate research by Dr. Pai's team also demonstrated exactly how long it took to diagnose TB correctly in India on average: nearly sixty days, and three different doctors.[6] From the time symptoms appeared to the time a patient was correctly diagnosed, patients went to informal and private sectors, especially pharmacists, and formal providers before eventually ending up in government hospitals once they ran out of money.

"It is a long, complex pathway—uniformly across the country. India's TB care is a leaky cascade, with patients falling through the cracks at every stage," Dr. Pai told me when I interviewed him in April 2019. Every day they are not diagnosed, a TB patient's symptoms worsen. And they could infect people around them.

As the illness gets worse, families get frantic, experimenting with any cure that may help, including outright magical remedies like goat's milk and change of scenery, "cures" as unscientific as those from eighteenth-century America. Too often, by the time the patient has found the right doctor, the small cough has been treated by three different doctors with different cocktails of anti-biotics and most likely has morphed into a nasty drug-resistant strain of TB.

Tuberculosis has become the most lethal killer of all.

The Black Death, or bubonic plague, of the fourteenth century is considered the greatest of all plagues. After the dust settled, it was responsible for fifty million deaths around the world.[7] TB, conservatively, kills that many people every three decades.

And we are nowhere near ready to fight its current bloodcurdling antibiotic-resistant avatar.

In India, the worst-affected country in the world, a patient with the milder version, drug-sensitive tuberculosis, has a 50 percent chance of successfully completing treatment. If the patient has DR TB, the odds are stacked against her. There is a 10 percent chance of successfully completing a DR TB diagnosis.

Since only one in three suspected TB patients is correctly treated, the other two—overtreated, undertreated, and/or untreated—will infect ten to fifteen other people in their lifetime.

It is a pay-it-forward nightmare.

Each study since 1991, when Udwadia found his first DR TB patient, shows that India's policy has piled one error on top of another, but the through line is that a significant majority of India's private doctors have never known how to diagnose or treat TB patients correctly. They have also been reluctant to refer them to other doctors who might know better.

"Our data shows public sector does better and yet people still prefer private hospitals," Dr. Udwadia summarized bluntly for the audience in the conference hall.

The scale of the problem is clear: India's private sector doctors outnumber public sector doctors thirteen to one. Between 50 to

70 percent of Indian TB patients go to the private sector for treatment and diagnosis, where they are treated "without science, and without compassion" in the words of Dr. Pai. Almost 75 percent of patients buy expensive TB drugs in the private market rather than go to a government hospital, where the drugs are free.

Indian patients choose expensive, faulty private sector care largely because of social snobbery. India's government-run hospitals cater to poor patients—most of them from the lower caste and lower class. Anyone with viable options, which is to say money, almost always prefers somewhere else.

The government hospitals are overworked, understaffed, and underfunded, and the doctors are often exhausted, brusque, and tough talking as a result. They do not advertise compassion, but they are medically sound, not having an incentive to over- or undertreat patients.

Dr. Udwadia studied the reasons people didn't like government hospitals. He asked two hundred patients why they came to an expensive private sector doctor like himself when the government hospitals in Mumbai would treat them free of cost.

He told me that the patients' answers ranged from "rude staff," "uncaring doctors," "no privacy," "inflexible hospital timing," and "long distances" to simply saying the hospitals did not treat patients with dignity. "While the government clinics are free, it is the kind of free no one can afford," reflected Dr. Udwadia.

Unable to get the private sector to volunteer reliable TB data, in 2012, the Indian government declared TB a notifiable disease—115 years after New York City had made TB a notifiable disease in 1897.

That meant private doctors were obligated to report to the government every case of TB they treated.

India's self-regulated private hospitals simply ignored the new law.

For six years, the government tried and failed to implement the order, as things steadily got worse. In 2018, the government passed another notification, making the nonreporting of tuberculosis a punishable offence, with a jail term of up to two years. At the same time, Prime Minister Narendra Modi announced that India would end TB by 2025, on a "mission mode" and five years ahead of the Sustainable Development Goal deadline of 2030.

True to character, Modi treated the public health issue as a law-and-order problem. "It used to amuse me earlier, now it makes me angry," said Dr. Udwadia during an interview at his office in Hinduja Hospital. "The government tried to enforce notification, including with jail terms; private hospitals *still* don't notify. The small private clinics won't get on the phone to notify the government every time they get a TB patient. All official figures are *considerable* underestimates. Even now, the number of TB patients in this country is a huge underestimation by at least 1.5 million cases."

The people who have eyes to see what is unfolding see a continual eruption of a deadly disease on a scale never witnessed before. A world we assumed belonged to the past, one in which a pathogen could wipe out a generation as doctors helplessly watched, is very much a present reality in India. And its consequences are not limited to India.

Scientifically speaking, the TB bacterium is an evolutionary masterpiece. It must constantly evolve—mutate—to survive.

Having lived with us for centuries, the TB bacillus has become an expert in seamlessly jumping species, say, for example, from cows to humans, adapting each time. Like any master mutator, it has become increasingly difficult to kill.

The doctors working in Mumbai's TB clinics witness an unfolding nightmare. Listening to doctors talk about antibiotic resistance is like hearing characters in a horror movie as they navigate increasingly limited options.

One doctor joked about being at that point in the film when you realize the call is coming from inside your own house.

* * *

After a forty-year drought, two new antibiotics to treat TB became available toward the end of 2012. Johnson & Johnson got accelerated approval for bedaquiline in 2012, which proved to be fast and effective. The WHO now recommends bedaquiline for all drug-resistant patients. Two years later delamanid was approved. It was equally impressive.

Following promising clinical trial results, delamanid received accelerated approval because it was urgently needed. Patients like Piya need both drugs, and WHO recommends that governments make them available free of charge through national programs.

In India, you cannot walk over to the nearest chemist and purchase these drugs. They are not available over the counter. The patient must *qualify*. This is a nerve-wracking process during which patients compete to get lifesaving medicines.

To be considered an ideal candidate, you must be just sick enough, not too sick or too far gone in the illness for the government to "waste" new medicine on you, and not too simple a case either. In technical terms, you have to be pre-XDR or XDR.

In real life this means, as a government policy, the drug is available to patients who are a half step from death.

Once qualified, the patient must wait for the wheels of Indian bureaucracy to turn. The government provides paperwork certifying patients as bona fide TB cases. To make this Kafkaesque hell a little more challenging for patients who are already fighting for their lives, the Indian government approved delamanid and bedaquiline to be used in a pilot project across multiple cities, none overlapping.[8] While bedaquiline is in short supply, delamanid is completely unavailable outside of these six sites.

By conservative estimates, the Indian government maintains there are 147,000 DR TB patients who qualify for new therapies. Most need both drugs; very few can get either. In December 2019, 9,415 patients had been prescribed bedaquiline and 353 delamanid.[9] As a result, the outbreak of XDR TB is snowballing.

Dr. Udwadia had initially refused to take Piya on as a patient. He doesn't take many pediatric cases because they will need drugs that he can prescribe but patients won't be able to access.

It is a lost cause; doctors get heartsore from such defeats.

He eventually took Piya's case partly because it exemplified the struggles of hundreds of thousands of Indian TB patients. Piya was the poster child of a failing health system, and Dr. Udwadia wanted the whole country, and indeed the world, to know about her.

In April 2019, Piya greeted me in her apartment in Mumbai and then quickly darted into the kitchen. When she came back, she was balancing a tray in her hand with some biscuits and a glass of water on it. She was mostly silent as her parents talked about the last year of their lives, about how it all had become about her.

For an eleven-year-old, Piya sat in an unusually ladylike posture. She didn't slump into the sofa but eased into it, back straight, head up, knees closed, and hands resting on her thigh.

In the last year, Piya had had to grow up in a hurry, and her younger sibling, at eight, had had to grow up even faster. Her sister helped dress her wounds, cared for her when their parents were absent, carried the bedpans, and helped clean up. Alia, her mother, quit her job to take care of the family.

In November 2018, Piya "fell down, hurt herself on the same ankle." The family had gone to a birthday party, a rare family outing, Alia adds, in a tone familiar to most parents. "I was away for a second to put something in a trash can. When I came back, Piya kept saying she was sorry for falling down, over and over again."

By this time, Piya had been on delamanid for six months.

The drug treatment meant that Piya did not need any more debridement surgeries, but there were many side effects to the antibiotics. Her teeth changed color and turned yellowish. Her skin itched and flushed red, as if she had applied a thin layer of kumkum (vermillion) on her face. There were other reactions as well: nausea from the drugs, stomachache, fever, fatigue, and loss of appetite.

Piya's family had no clue about this when the treatment had begun. Indeed, the family's first reaction to a diagnosis of TB was relief: "When we heard it was TB, we thought at least it is curable. We were praying that it should not be rheumatic arthritis," said her father, thinking back to when they were still trying to find out what was causing her to limp.

But when they tested Piya for drug sensitivity—testing how many antibiotic drugs her body responded to—it was clear that Piya was XDR. All the available types of antibiotics were ineffective on her.

"Whatever drugs we were giving Piya since March were useless for her," Alia recalled.

"Why the doctors started Piya on first and second line of drugs before getting the drug sensitivity tests (DST) back, we do not know," her father wondered, spelling out one of the biggest complaints TB patients have with private doctors in India: treating before they know what they are treating.

This simple step—putting patients on varying cocktails of antibiotics without a DST—is a major cause of the increase in antibiotic resistance.

The first time Piya's family heard the term "XDR TB" was when the DST test result came back, plunging them into medical research—WebMD, books, calling doctors they knew. They pulled every string a middle-class Indian family could.

"Our doctor told us she could not treat 'such kind of patients.' That's when we realized Piya had one of the most difficult-to-treat superbugs, and it was on the ankle joint. The doctors told us we had limited options," her father remembered.

The family was starting to panic, dress-rehearsing tragedy, like most of us do when we feel doomed. Piya's parents felt utterly helpless as they stood over their sleeping child, haunted by every possible tragic scenario.

In just a few days, their lives had been upended.

Everything was fine. Then, one day their daughter was walking with a limp.

Before they knew it, the family was fighting to get access to medicines, without which the disease would likely kill Piya. It wasn't until two weeks after the dramatic trip to Tokyo, in May 2018, when the family was granted access to a six months' supply of delamanid that they could slow down to process what they were going through—after they had put Piya on a viable treatment plan. A typical XDR TB patient is in treatment for around two years.

Piya's father was planning a second trip to Tokyo to beg Otsuka officials for another six months of drugs, once again on compassionate grounds, when he was told that the compassionate exception was a one-time event. If Piya was to get a further supply of delamanid, it would have to come from the Médecins Sans Frontières (MSF) clinic in Mumbai instead.

Expecting Indian families to go to Tokyo and appeal to the pharmaceutical company or aid organizations like MSF is a cruel policy and one that, for practical reasons, excludes the majority of TB sufferers in India.

The government's callousness turns families into experts on subjects ranging from antibiotic resistance to patent law and drug development as they try to argue and convince the health departments of their right to access newer medicines.

"How many fathers can do it?" Piya's father asked. He petitioned the health ministry and Janssen Pharmaceuticals, the American pharmaceutical giant Johnson & Johnson subsidiary that owns bedaquiline.

For a few months, the company, and the Indian health ministry, told the family that Piya was at the top of the priority list. Once the government approved the case, Janssen would grant them access.

But nothing happened.

"The government never replied. The company stopped replying as well. I got to know from Dr. Udwadia's office that Piya was rejected," her father said. "It makes me angry. This drug is available for free in other countries. I pay taxes here. My government has done nothing to help me and is instead rationing drugs that can save life."

By the time the family was told that bedaquiline had been refused to Piya, they were all in various stages of exhaustion.

The family's finances were seriously depleted from the trips to hospitals and Tokyo, the strain had affected all their relationships, and they still did not have the steady supply of drugs they needed.

Through all this, one question hovered over the parents like a deadly miasma: Where did Piya, who only goes to school and comes back home, pick up this dangerous disease? Where did she get XDR TB?

The truth is, in Mumbai, it could be anywhere—on overcrowded buses and trains, in movie theaters, or in the streets where men spit and people cough and sneeze without shielding. No one is insulated from TB. Once acquired, the bacteria will lie low if you have a healthy immune system—even for decades—before it starts multiplying inside.

Coping with this stigma has not been easy.

Even though Piya has a noninfectious kind of TB (in the ankle bone and not in the lungs), the full weight of her classmates' ignorance has been brought to bear upon her.

Conversations with Piya move seamlessly from preteen concerns to emotionally heavy and deeply introspective statements. "I learnt in biology about tissues. When we get cut on our hand, something called platelets forms a clotting layer on the skin," she told me.

Mentioning TB for the first time, she says, "Sometimes my teacher says the word 'TB' and I freeze. I think she knows. I am always scared people will find out."

"What will happen if they find out?"

"They will call me sick girl. I'll be the girl with TB."

"Did someone say that to you?"

At this point, Alia steps in.

"Her complexion turned dark because of the antibiotics. So, she looks red, and her friends make fun of it. Her teeth turned yellow, again because of the toxicity of the antibiotics. Her friends told her to clean her teeth."

It broke the parents' hearts, and they again asked the doctors for help, only to realize this was the least of the doctors' concerns. Her parents told Piya to keep calm and explain to her friends that it was a side effect of her medication.

The family went through many unspoken miseries, and four doctors, before they arrived at Dr. Udwadia's clinic. It had taken more than sixty days, and by then Piya had developed DR TB.

* * *

Piya's treatment should have been straightforward. The government ran a TB center in Khar, close to where Piya's family lived in Mumbai. Ideally, that's the one-stop shop for TB patients in the neighborhood, unless they require tertiary care. But the center told Piya to go to Sewri TB Hospital, Asia's largest TB hospital, overwhelming it needlessly.

There was no way her parents were taking Piya there. Sewri is, in Alia's words, "not for the weakhearted."

The one time she went, she saw a young girl with TB in the brain. "That kid was my daughter's age. The doctors had admitted her, but they did not have drugs to treat her. The patients, sometimes young kids, were just waiting to die," adds Alia in a breathless rebuke of the system.

Initially, the family went to Hinduja Hospital to see a different doctor. When they got to the hospital, Piya's father barged into Dr. Udwadia's clinic. He believes it saved Piya's life because it was Dr. Udwadia who persuaded the family to go to Tokyo.

"We had the money, so we could go to Tokyo. If we didn't have money, we would also be crowding some TB clinic in Mumbai, like thousands of other families. Do the government officials not realize that they are forcing patients with regular TB to develop MDR and XDR TB when they deny us medicines? Any other country would treat patients for free—until they are completely cured—so as to not infect other people in the city."

It need not be this way.

Piya's family was clear about what India should do: "If I have a prescription from a doctor, I should get the medicine at our neighborhood TB clinic, for free. The government clinics need to start treating patients with dignity," Piya's father declared.

Much like containing a wildfire, when you diagnose DR TB correctly, and patients are put on correct antibiotics, it is equivalent to creating a firebreak. There is still smoke and heat, but the spread has been interrupted, wildfire contained.

Ultimately, Piya was able to get enough treatment to recover from XDR TB. She was lucky; her family was affluent and intrepid, and she survived. She has begun to plan for a future that a few months earlier she dared not dream might ever be hers.

"I want to become a lawyer and fight for TB patients to have access to medicines." If she follows through, there is a good chance that thousands of poor Indians will need her services, because TB is not going away on its own.

That's simply not what it does.

The history of tuberculosis medicine, at its base, is a story of science's battle to keep pace with the bacteria's evolution.

Professor Jennifer Furin, who teaches at Harvard Medical School, has long been saying that India's TB crisis is the world's problem. If India does not modernize its antiquated TB policy and get a grip on its TB epidemic, it will be bad news not only for India but also for the rest of the world.

It is an airborne respiratory disease, and global travel spreads it, no matter how many walls—of privilege, race, caste, and class—we create. Western countries where TB is no longer an epidemic demand chest x-rays from Indians before granting them visas as a precautionary measure. But they don't screen returning Westerners who may also have been exposed to TB.

In that way, India's antibiotic apocalypse is on the move.

CHAPTER 7

———— ◆ ————

SHREYA

For every patient like Piya, who gets on treatment despite the odds, there are thousands who do not, despite their heroic efforts and the sacrifices of their families.

Shreya Tripathi, a young girl I never had a chance to meet, belongs to the pantheon of teenage girls who fight to change the world: Malala Yousafzai. Greta Thunberg. Emma González.

Unlike her contemporaries—who shook the collective conscious and brought global attention to important causes—Shreya died trying. Her story barely registered on the collective conscious of the country she lived in. It should have, but India is a crowded country, and tragedies get lost in a country where tragedies are piled on tragedies every single day.

She suffered from XDR TB but was denied bedaquiline by her doctors and the Indian health ministry. The government, the ultimate custodian of the nation's health, asked her to go home and die. She challenged the decision, took her case to court, and won.

Her victory was Pyrrhic. She died in October 2018, and the country's officialdom wanted to bury her story with her.[1]

December 20, 2016, was one of those winter mornings in Delhi when everything is enveloped in the smog of chronic air pollution. On that day, in one of Delhi High Court's crowded courtrooms, lawyers, activists, and press had gathered for an extraordinary case. Shreya's father, Krishna Tripathi, had filed a civil writ petition on behalf of his sixteen-year-old daughter. Shreya was too sick to do so herself.

The family had endured a juggernaut of injustices.

By 2016, Shreya had been suffering from XDR TB—amplified by wrong treatment—for four years. She was in urgent need of bedaquiline. Everyone involved knew there was a small chance of success. Shreya was running out of time, and the family had to do something.

Her family believed that she had been exposed to TB at school. She went through the same maze, the leaky cascade through which patients fall, that Dr. Pai and Dr. Udwadia have documented in study after study.

It took Shreya nearly four years to find Dr. Udwadia.

Shreya was initially treated by a private doctor in Patna, Bihar, where she lived. Like Piya, she was also put on TB treatment without a DST, so it was only "a few months later" that her family discovered Shreya was resistant to the first line of drugs. And the second, after which "the disease spread relentlessly," her father recalled.[2] The family had wasted an entire year searching for a correct diagnosis. By September 2013, her family knew she had MDR TB. After repeatedly failing to respond to antibiotics prescribed by her private doctor, she landed at the government hospital, also in Bihar.

She was then treated for MDR TB by the government doctors, once again without a comprehensive DST.

Without it, doctors were flying blind. They did not know what antibiotics worked on her, so they carpet-bombed her body—the medical version of the common "spray and pray" marketing technique.

There was, unsurprisingly, no improvement in her condition.

Watching her deteriorate by the day, her father turned to the Vallabhbhai Patel Chest Institute in New Delhi, one of the country's best super-specialty TB hospitals. The Chest Institute referred her to a bigger, tertiary care, government-run center: Lala Ram Swarup Institute of Tuberculosis and Respiratory Diseases, or LRS TB Hospital.

It is among India's biggest TB hospitals, located in Delhi.

For the next six months, the family lost more precious time as a battery of tests was repeated. The confirmatory tests, especially the DST, took weeks and cost Shreya the only thing she did not have: time.

They finally confirmed, as was already blindingly obvious, that Shreya was resistant to the most powerful anti-TB drugs—fluoroquinolones (ofloxacin) and injectables (capreomycin, kanamycin, etc.).

She had XDR TB because of the varying cocktails she had been prescribed.

Once it was apparent to the LRS doctors that the poorly designed treatment plan was responsible for her XDR TB, they washed their hands of Shreya's case. Dr. Rupak Singla, head of the department of TB at LRS Hospital, advised that her treatment be stopped. The doctors abruptly withheld the medicines and informed the family that there was no hope.

In desperation, the family started searching for their next option, and that is how they ended up at Dr. Udwadia's clinic, finally finding the doctor they'd been looking for since 2012.

When Dr. Udwadia reviewed Shreya's medical files, he told the family to "try hard" to get bedaquiline as a salvage therapy.

In Shreya's case, getting a bedaquiline prescription meant Dr. Udwadia had to either arrange for the drug from the pharmaceutical company (like he had for Piya) or send her back to government-run hospitals like LRS in the hope that she would receive treatment without delay.

In 2016—four years after bedaquiline was approved—it was still available only at six government hospitals across India. Shreya's family could not go to Tokyo, which meant they were back in Delhi, in the office of the same doctors at LRS Hospital who had already turned them away once.

When she went back specifically to ask for bedaquiline, the doctors once again turned her down, saying the drug was only available to patients who lived in Delhi.

To critics of the Indian government's policy, this rationing of much-needed medication is a human rights violation, one that future generations will look back on in shock and disbelief. It is unforgivable that a country the size of India designed a TB policy that delivers an essential drug like bedaquiline only to someone who lives (1) in one of the five cities where the government was running a pilot project and (2) within a five-kilometer radius of the government hospitals.

The policy, instead of being dictated by science, was dictated by arbitrary, unscientific, and cruel restrictions, designed to exclude vulnerable patients and to minimize India's official TB numbers.

In countries like India, where patients are not entitlement literate (not aware of their rights) and usually trusting of authority, most patients believe that *they* are at fault—for being poor or living too far or being too sick—or that they are being punished because of their karma.

That's the circle of hell Shreya's family found themselves in when they went back to LRS, condemned.

When Shreya was at LRS, Dr. Singla (the same doctor who had told the Tripathi family there was no hope eighteen months earlier) now recommended more tests, more sputum samples, another DST—all of which the family undertook. It is unclear what Singla expected the tests to show, given that everyone already knew Shreya had XDR TB.

The family agreed, and new tests were done, at a typically leisurely pace.

For the next two months, Shreya's father kept calling the hospital for the test results. His daughter was dying, and the hospital kept asking him to wait. Eventually, when they called him back with results, it was more bad news: the sample had been contaminated; there were no reliable findings. The tests that were *not needed* had not been done properly, and it had cost the family two months. The hospital, once again, wanted samples and requested the family to wait for fresh, hopefully uncontaminated results.

The family complied once again.

In December 2016, Shreya provided a fresh sample for even more tests. She was asked to wait another four to six weeks for the results.

At that point Shreya knew she could not afford to wait any longer. "I told Papa to go to court. Even if it's too late for me, at least other patients will benefit from it. Just imagine how hard it must be for really poor people to get this drug," she told the *Guardian*.[3]

She wanted her suffering to have meaning.

That's how the family landed at the crowded courtroom in Delhi High Court on the smog-filled winter morning of December

20, 2016, in the fifth year of Shreya's TB diagnosis, after she had failed *five rounds* of toxic anti-TB treatment.

The medicines had ravaged her body. She had to stop going to school and was confined to a wheelchair. The eighteen-year-old weighed twenty-five kilograms. Her government had effectively left her alone to struggle with pulmonary XDR, a deadly, virulent infection, for five full years.

As the family went to court in December 2016, Shreya's case hit the headlines around the world. India's problem with drug-resistant tuberculosis was becoming too huge to be swept under the carpet of empty political rhetoric.

Professor Furin was keenly following the developments from Harvard: "Some colleague mentioned about this young woman in India who could not get bedaquiline." Furin told her colleague, "Lemme know if you want me to help."

Her friend in India replied almost immediately, saying, "Actually there is something you may be able to do. Would you mind if we put you in touch with Shreya's lawyers?"

The friend connected Furin with Anand Grover from Lawyers Collective, a prominent not-for-profit legal aid organization with an established record of defending human rights in India. The group of lawyers specialize in issues relating to women's rights and the rights of India's HIV and LGBTQ communities.

Grover was representing Shreya in court and wanted Professor Furin's medical opinion on the scientific claims about bedaquiline. He asked her to take a look at the testimonies submitted by the Indian doctors to see if they were in line with WHO recommendations and global best practices.

When she looked at what the Indian government was claiming, Professor Furin was astonished at the flagrant deceitfulness.

"The doctors were saying blatantly untrue things in the testimony. Shreya had a test that documented she was XDR TB from several months prior. But the doctors were saying that even though Shreya has documented resistance to the injectables, the floroquinalones, etc.—she still needed to prove, once more, for the court that she had XDR."

Professor Furin explained this to Shreya's lawyer by comparing it to doctors demanding fresh tests from cancer patients to prove repeatedly that they still had cancer—while withholding treatment. "I told Anand [Grover] if she had XDR TB before, and had been unsuccessfully treated for it, it's not like the disease will somehow go away. You don't go from having XDR TB to getting treated and staying sick and then to *not* having XDR TB. Usually, at that point, you have even more resistance."

Grover asked if she would formally submit her opinion on Harvard Medical School letterhead paper.

Several of the statements from the LRS Hospital doctors made no sense to Professor Furin. "India's government frequently tries to explain away the great injustice they perpetrated against this young girl. Sometimes, they hide behind a meaningless scientific facade, claiming there was not enough medical evidence to give Shreya the drug. Most often, they cloak themselves in the respected mantle of public health and talk about preventing the development of resistance to this precious medication and how they need to 'protect' bedaquiline—in case people need it in the future. They almost never mention how they failed to protect Shreya, whose life depended on receiving bedaquiline as soon as possible."

In other countries with a high incidence of TB, bedaquiline and delamanid are more easily available.[4]

"Anytime someone says they need to protect the drug, I say, for whom? I have patients who line up at my clinic every single day. Would you like me to tell them that I cannot give them medicine right now because somebody else might need it in the future?" Furin said.

Professor Furin found it incomprehensible that India—a country known for having highly trained medical doctors—was questioning the science behind bedaquiline. "This is not a country where doctors are working with minimum training and rudimentary research. In India, we don't have to train or explain to doctors about clinical research. But, when it came to bedaquiline, people only wanted to interpret the science to back up their point. They were convinced they didn't want this drug. So, they twisted the science," she told me over Skype in April 2019.

She knew from her experience of working in India that doctors didn't always back science. In July 2015, a year and a half before Shreya's court case, Professor Furin had visited India to conduct a workshop jointly held by WHO and USAID on bedaquiline. "They were supposed to be putting together a plan to scale up bedaquiline in India. There were a lot of misstatements. It was one of the most frustrating workshops I had ever been to in my whole life. There were many, many Indian doctors who supported using the drug. A large majority of people in that room wanted access to this drug. But there were five or six people who kept saying no, no, no. It tanked the whole thing. I was surprised by it, and I remember thinking, it is going to be an uphill battle to get doctors to use this drug in India."

The government questioned the data, the clinical trials, regulatory approval for the drug—just about every aspect of it.

To Furin, it was "a bullshit argument. The first drug to ever be tested against MDR TB and showing results against drug-resistant TB, and they don't want to prescribe it? I don't understand the logic of it."

After Shreya died, Professor Furin wrote, "Instead of protecting her, the RNTCP [India's national TB program] forced Shreya—who was fighting for her life—to have to spend some of her last days on earth fighting against the formidable bureaucracy."[5] With some distance from the litigation, and with time to have reflected on what happened, Professor Furin felt that many doctors had a "bad feeling" toward patients. "They say things like patients won't take it, 'they' don't listen to us. 'They' will just create more resistance. This idea of not trusting the patients who come to them for help when they are sick—and instead viewing them as dangerous people who will ruin the drug for everybody—there is a lot of that type of distrust."

None of that is new or limited to India or to TB.

"This is as racist as saying Africans cannot get antiretroviral drugs because they cannot tell the time. This notion of protecting the medicine for an 'unnamed other' instead of giving it to someone in front of you is morally fraught," insisted Professor Furin, referring to a European Commission hearing in Brussels from September 2000.

It was a time when the HIV epidemic was spreading fast. Celebrities were singing for Africa, raising money for AIDS awareness, while the expensive HIV drugs were locked in patents.

Most African nations did not have access to newly developed HIV therapies at that time. There was an international debate among developed nations about giving access to HIV medicines to African patients. The argument against doing so was that patients in Africa would misuse medicines and develop resistance. This resistance, and mutated new strains of HIV, would come back and kill Americans or Europeans.

"During the HIV epidemic, the HIV activists worked together, and this narrative was shot down pretty quickly. They called BS on it. In TB, it is allowed to persist," Professor Furin noted.

"Inherent in that question is the fact that infectious diseases that affect poor people could someday affect rich people—or white people. Instead of disproportionately affecting poorer people, with darker skin, we, the rich and the white, want to save these medicines for *us*, for *later*. No one comes out and says it, but that's what is inherent in that argument," Furin concluded.

Furin has been interviewed extensively in the Indian media, calling out the Indian government on its policy of drug rationing. Throughout, she has consistently maintained that the drugs are being saved for the rich: "Whichever doctor says we need to protect the drug definitely doesn't see patients. If they see patients, they don't like their patients. There is no way that conversation ends with anything other than an admission of classism and racism."

It is hard to disagree with Professor Furin's piercing judgment.

By restricting access to bedaquiline, the Indian government buried Shreya, her family, and many other patients like her, in paperwork. It was death by red tape, bureaucracy at its ruthless best, serving to protect a patented drug owned by an American pharmaceutical company.

But before I dive into why black and brown patients, such as Piya and Shreya, have their fates sealed by people they cannot see, according to rules they do not know, we need to talk about a man called Jim Logan.

* * *

The first podcast ever was recorded in 1996, or so Logan claims. It was a low-tech, crude version of what we now know and consisted of a ninety-minute recording of a woman reading out articles.

It was a kind of audio magazine.

Jim Logan had made the tape while toying with an idea. He envisioned a future in which anything you wanted to listen to— music, newspaper reports, and so forth—could be downloaded to your electronic device.

It was a neat idea: a digital music player that would automatically update with new episodes based on your preferences, the same way as Netflix algorithms would later work. But the idea failed. Logan never made any money from it. In fact, he claims to have lost around $1.6 million.

His young company, PersonalAudio Inc., soon went under.

That cassette, however, of the woman reading out a magazine, became the epicenter of a litigation marathon that threatened everyone who has ever made a podcast or listened to one. The cassette would make Logan the world's most infamous "patent troll."

A patent, granted by the government, gives an inventor, a company, or an individual a twenty-year legal monopoly over the sale of their product. Patent *trolling* is when someone who does not necessarily have a product somehow establishes a patent on the idea.

It happens frequently. Trolls make an indecent amount of money seeking damages from competitors who infringe, as they see it, on their bona fide patents.

A second way to troll is to take an already existing idea— something that is already in use—and establish a patent on it as an "emerging technology." For example, if the first person who made a chicken nugget got a patent on it, *only* that person is legally allowed to make chicken nuggets for the duration of the patent—twenty years. Given the implication of granting a twenty-year monopoly, logic would dictate that patents be granted after careful consideration by governments.

But that's not how the patent system works.

In 2000, the US Patent Office granted a patent to a man for toasted bread.[6] He claimed to have stumbled upon a new "bread refreshing method." Historically, patent ownership seems to bring out the worst in all of us.

An English scientist, Henry Talbot, thought he owned photography.[7] He was the holder of a patent that affected the early development of commercial photography in Britain. While everywhere else in the world people were simply buying the apparatus and using it, in Britain, only people he chose, and those who paid him money, could use photography. Thomas Edison thought he owned Kinetograph, a first-generation movie camera, and, by extension, movies.[8] In 1898, Edison sued American Mutoscope and Biograph Pictures, claiming that the studio had infringed on his patent.

Since then, free market capitalism and intellectual property laws have only made ownership of words, symbols, smells, designs, creative content, and existing knowledge worse.

Candy Crush trademarked the English word "saga" because they had a few games with that word at the end. Apple thinks it owns rounded edges on rectangular phones. They successfully sued Samsung, setting off a "smartphone patent war" in America. On May 2, 2014, Samsung was instructed to pay US$119.6 million to Apple for patent violations.

There is a lot of money in patents.

Legally speaking, the first person to stamp a patent on an idea— to *write* it down and get the government to grant a patent—has ownership over it. This is not always the person who *had* the original idea. Essentially, the patent system is broken and difficult to navigate, and therefore most patent litigations end in settlements.

Stories of patent-like programs can be found as far back as 500 BC, in an ancient Greek city called Sybaris.[9] It is widely accepted that the first informal patent system was adopted in Renaissance Italy. Venetian glass blowers were granted monopolies when they migrated to other areas of Europe to protect their skills against those of local workers and to preserve Venice's lucrative glassblowing industry. The first patent granted in the United States was in 1790.

Patents stimulate interest in research and development (R&D) by protecting the efforts of new researchers and innovators. But not always.

Before Jim Logan's company went belly-up, he wrote down his idea, drew some pictures to describe it, and acquired a patent on a vague proto-podcast notion. The exact words he used were "an audio program and a messaging distribution system." The language was sufficiently imprecise that for a brief while, Logan interpreted it to mean he owned podcasts.

The first company that suffered significantly because of the patent system's flaw when it comes to vaguely asserted patents was Apple.

Logan had sat on his podcast patent for the next fourteen years, until he sued Apple in 2009 for two patent infringements.[10] He said they owed him money, as they had been using his idea, despite the fact that Logan had nothing to do with the creation of downloadable playlists or iPods or the technology that edited the audio for podcasts. Logan won $8 million. Apple appealed, and the two sides eventually settled, as invariably happens with patent litigations. Encouraged by his settlement, Logan went after other industry giants like Samsung, Amazon, CBS, and NBC and settled with them as well.

After he was done suing the big fish, Logan came after the small ones.

He started sending successful podcasters letters asking them to pay him. He wasn't suing the people who made the laptop or the microphone. He was suing the end user who bought the technology, used it, and made a podcast. By 2013, Logan was sending threatening legal letters to popular podcasters like comedian Marc Maron, who was making a comedy podcast called *WTF*. Maron didn't run a big business, let alone a multinational corporation. He was a guy who had bought a laptop and a microphone and made the podcast in his garage.

The patent system is a rich man's game. It is expensive to get a patent. It is even more expensive to challenge a patent. In general, podcasters don't make a lot of money, and a patent litigation, like the one faced by Maron, could bankrupt people. Logan sent out similar letters to podcaster Adam Carolla and HowStuffWorks, another popular podcast.

Logan never used podcasting technology himself, never made one, never intended to. He did not even listen to podcasts, according to an interview with NPR from May 2013.[11] He simply wanted a licensing fee: a tax that small-time podcasters, working out of their garages, had to cough up if they wanted to continue podcasting.

He generally didn't specify what fee he wanted; the defendant had to make an offer.

He was quietly profiting from the creativity of others or threatening to shut them down. Patent trolling has become so much of a nuisance that Broadcast.com founder Mark Cuban and Minecraft creator Markus Persson donated $500,000 to the Electronic Frontier Foundation (EFF), a leading nonprofit organization defending civil liberties in the digital world, to endow Mark Cuban's chair to "Eliminate Stupid Patents."[12] The EFF thought Logan's patent was stupid and fought it, successfully. They launched a campaign to "Save Podcasting" back in 2013 to raise funds for the legal battle and to find earlier examples of the same method of creating and distributing content.[13] The legal strategy was simple. EFF went looking for anyone who had made a podcast—an audio recording program—before October 2, 1996, the day Logan had filed his patent.

Of course, someone had.

So, EFF proved successfully that Logan wasn't the first one to make such a recording. Jim Logan did not do any of the hard work. He had done no inventing. For ten years, brilliant people at Apple worked hard to bring to market the software we use every day: iPods, iTunes, and podcasts.

Patents are so foundational to the American way of life that they find mention in the Constitution, "to promote useful arts and sciences." Tragically, some patents now do the exact opposite of what they intended to do: they stifle invention.

Logan is the destructive side of the great American invention story.

And his story is essential because you cannot understand how pharmaceutical patents work without understanding technological patents. There are two reasons for this: One, new drugs, vaccines, and diagnostics are first and foremost new technologies.

And two, Bill Gates.

Without patent protection for Windows and other Microsoft products, Bill Gates would certainly not be among the world's richest men. He would not be poor by any stretch, but he would not have a billion-dollar fortune without the monopolies on his software. Understandably, he is an advocate of tighter patent protections.

However, back in 1991, Bill Gates sang a different tune on patents. In a memo to his senior executives, he wrote, "If people had understood how patents would be granted when most of today's ideas were invented, and had taken out patents, the industry would be at a complete standstill today." He worried that "some large company will patent some obvious thing" and use the patent to "take as much of our profits as they want."[14] This memo was written when Microsoft was a growing company, challenging entrenched incumbents like IBM and Novell. It had only eight patents to its name. Recognizing the threat to his company, Gates initiated an aggressive patenting program. Today Microsoft holds more than fifty-nine thousand patents, and Gates is one of the loudest voices promoting patent protections.

But the Bill Gates of 1991 was right, especially about how patents apply to the pharmaceutical industry.

Patent laws are not international treaties; they are national laws based on the needs of the country. Global trade organizations (like the World Trade Organization) provide flexibilities for countries to issue patents, or revoke them, based on their needs.

One of the most effective uses of this flexibility was by the American government, a week after 9/11, when five anthrax-laced letters were dropped in a mailbox in Trenton, New Jersey, on September 18, 2001. Those envelopes, with their payloads, were sent to news outlets including NBC, CBS, ABC, the *New York Post*, and the *National Enquirer*. By October, America was gripped in anthrax panic as it claimed the first victim, Robert Stevens, a photo editor in a company that owned the *Sun* and *Enquirer*.

The only anti-anthrax treatment, Cipro (or Ciprofloxacin), was under a patent in the US until 2003, owned by the German pharmaceutical company Bayer. No other drug company was allowed to commercially manufacture and/or sell the generic versions of this drug in the US until Bayer's patent expired, except under extraordinary circumstances. The Bush administration said it would cite the "public health emergency" clause, threatening to issue a compulsory license (CL) and suspend Bayer's patent—allowing affordable generic drugs to be made so the US could stockpile in case of widespread anthrax exposure.

The CL would allow the US government to purchase Cipro from manufacturers other than Bayer, driving down prices. In addition, under US law, the government was exempt from paying any compensation to Bayer for suspending its patent.[15]

Just five Americans had died, and thirty-one people in the US Capitol had tested positive for anthrax exposure. Yet for a moment, Americans could not access lifesaving medicine cheaply and at scale, and a patent was perceived to be a threat to the health of the nation.

In contrast, when the HIV epidemic hit, millions of patients died, unable to access medicines that were locked under patents by American multinationals.

The first HIV drug, AZT (or azido-thymidine), was originally developed in 1964 by Jerome Horowitz, a US researcher who thought it could help treat cancer. He worked at the National Cancer Institute, so the drug's initial cost of discovery was borne by American taxpayers. The drug flopped and was shelved until the HIV epidemic, when in 1985, AZT was tried as a therapy, and it worked. The British pharmaceutical company Burroughs-Wellcome held the patent for AZT until 2005. The company later merged with GlaxoSmithKline. Just before the patent was about to expire, GlaxoSmithKline said that the drug was better when used in combination with another drug as a cocktail. So, they filed for another patent—extending their monopoly by another twenty years—until 2017, using a strategy known as "evergreening."

One way or another, AZT was patented from 1963 to 2017.

The case of AZT demonstrates that, more often than not, the patent system neither rewards inventions nor benefits the discoverer; the inventor of AZT (Jerome Horowitz) was not the patent holder (GlaxoSmithKline) for the drug. The argument that patents promote invention needs to be finally and permanently discredited and abandoned.

Today, as Indian children like Piya and Shreya struggle to access medicines after being handed an XDR TB diagnosis, the impact of global patent laws on health insecurities cannot be missed.

In a global pandemic, deaths don't just happen—they are inflicted on people, sometimes legally. Accessing new-generation TB drugs in India is like a spin of the roulette wheel—utterly up to chance.

The moral dilemma here cannot be evaded: the drug, bedaquiline, is owned by an American corporation, and the demands of its shareholders determine the fate of millions of TB patients around the world. The drugs are rationed due to a false shortage created by locking them under patent monopolies.

The majority of dying patients are brown or black, while a significant number of patent owners are not.

The net effect is that drug patents are often not only unfair but also racist.

To add insult to injury, the story of how Johnson & Johnson acquired bedaquiline's patent might make even Jim Logan blush.

* * *

The story of bedaquiline's development is of a genuinely collective effort.

Janssen Pharmaceuticals (a subsidiary of Johnson & Johnson) discovered bedaquiline around 2002, but clinical trials were not complete until 2012, when the USFDA gave Johnson & Johnson accelerated approval to get the drug to market quickly—based on phase IIb data, a huge money saver for the company, permitted because the medical community was desperately in need of new antibiotics to treat DR TB.

Several of the phase I and II clinical trials—when the safety and efficacy of the drug is established before the drug's registration—were sponsored by public and philanthropic organizations such as the US National Institutes of Health, National Institute of Allergy and Infectious Diseases, and the TB Alliance.

The last stage of clinical trial—phase III—was done by research institutes and treatment providers, including national TB programs of India and South Africa, the countries with the highest burden of TB.[16]

One of the most common side effects of the previous (and often ineffective) TB treatment is that one in four patients go deaf. It is a fifty-year-old drug that would not get a marketing license if it were applied for today, in Dr. Udwadia's opinion.

In contrast, bedaquiline is a humane, effective alternative. If you can get it.

When the drug was in the development stage, Johnson & Johnson benefited from every single provision that exists to encourage R&D. (See tables 1 and 2 in the appendix on the tax benefits Johnson & Johnson received.)

In February 2019, MSF sent an open letter to Johnson & Johnson, urging the pharmaceutical corporation to drop the prices of bedaquiline so that countries around the world could access an affordable and sustainable supply.[17] MSF argued that bedaquiline was too important to be restricted by price alone and that the company that made it had already received vast amounts of taxpayer money for their research and testing efforts: "These public contributions warrant a common right to use that should ensure that bedaquiline is accessible to all TB patients who need it and to TB programmes worldwide, especially in TB high-burden countries. J&J's secondary patent application blatantly disregards public contributions to the development of the drug, and thus the secondary patent claim should be unequivocally rejected."[18]

Disregarding the dire need for the drug, Johnson & Johnson has claimed sole ownership of it, protected by their patent. As a result they have priced the drug aggressively in America—where taxpayers had heavily invested in R&D and now pay $30,000 for a six-month course.

In India, where Johnson & Johnson manufactures this drug at a fraction of the cost, and exports to the rest of the world, the drug is rationed to a point that leaves TB patients therapeutically destitute.

After the clinical trials were done, Johnson & Johnson filed patents in at least fifty-two countries with a high burden of TB cases.[19] They filed multiple patents in each country, which can broadly be divided into five types:

Type 1: patent on the compound
Type 2: patent on the method of use of the compound to treat MDR TB
Type 3: "method of use" patent to treat latent TB

Type 4: patent on the process to make bedaquiline

Type 5: patent on the end use product that will come to market

While not all the patent applications identified may be pursued and/or granted, the applications indicate the obstacles that TB patients of modest means face when they seek treatment.

Bedaquiline is expected to yield US$3.49 billion in sales by 2024.

As of December 2019, only 51,098 people worldwide had received bedaquiline, nearly 50.7 percent of whom have been treated in South Africa after the government negotiated a discounted price with the company.

India has no such agreement, even though the drug is manufactured there.

In December 2014, due to the growing chorus from public health organizations demanding lower drug prices, Johnson & Johnson announced a partnership with the US Agency for International Development (USAID) to make the drug available in developing nations. Under this agreement with USAID, Janssen announced they would donate $30 million worth of bedaquiline, over a four-year period—a fraction of the rebates and incentives they benefited from during its development.

India received the lion's share of these donations.

Janssen donated twenty thousand courses of bedaquiline, and Otsuka donated four hundred courses of delamanid. Besides this, the Indian government has made no other provision to secure an affordable supply—leaving Indian citizens at the mercy of the limited generosity of foreign corporations.

Because India depended on donations, there was never enough bedaquiline for India's needs, and the government had to ration the drugs, condemning patients like Shreya to a miserable end.

Despite the unconscionable loss of life each year, the Modi administration has been reluctant to issue a CL, citing a public health emergency as the Bush administration did after the anthrax attacks.

Outside of India, countries acquire bedaquiline through the Global Drug Facility or GDF—the WHO's TB arm based in Geneva, Switzerland, and the largest global provider of TB medicines, diagnostics, and laboratory supplies to governments around the world.

The GDF has negotiated a price of US$340 for a six-month course of treatment. Outside of the GDF, bedaquiline is priced at $3,000 for middle-income countries and $30,000 for high-income countries. This is known as "tiered pricing"—when different classes of buyers are charged different prices for the same product.

Professor Furin said this was a terrible strategy: "When Johnson & Johnson first came out with the tiered pricing model, the activist community said two things: don't do tiered pricing. Don't do donations. We begged them to not do that. They did both. Our demand is, like they did for antiretrovirals during the HIV epidemic, to bring the drug price down to a dollar a day."

Tiered pricing and donations are both strategies deployed by Big Pharma to quiet criticisms of their excessive pricing and patent monopolies. Both strategies are morally appalling.

Donations, in particular, can never replace fair pricing.

In October 2016, MSF refused to accept a donation of one million pneumonia vaccine doses from Pfizer. The refusal made international headlines.[20] MSF had been trying to get their hands on that vaccine, Prevnar 13, since it was introduced in 2009, but the price was too high. Yet, MSF would not accept donations, imperiling children who would have received the vaccines, in a principled stand against the extremely high cost of many vaccines. Jason Cone, MSF executive director, later explained his decision, saying,

> Free is not always better. Donations often involve numerous conditions and strings attached, including restrictions on which patient populations and what geographic areas are allowed to receive the benefits. . . . Donations are often used as a way to make others "pay up." By giving the pneumonia vaccine away for free, pharmaceutical corporations can use this as justification for why prices remain high for others, including other humanitarian organizations and developing countries that also can't afford the vaccine. . . . Critically, donation offers can disappear as quickly as they come. The donor has ultimate control over when and how they choose to give their products away, risking interruption of programs, should the company decide it's no longer to their advantage.[21]

He ended by saying, if Pfizer genuinely cared about children dying from pneumonia, it should lower the price of its lifesaving pneumonia vaccine to five dollars per child instead of picking and choosing donations.

For this exact reason, Johnson & Johnson preferred a donation model to bring bedaquiline into India. Running a national program in a country the size of India, exclusively on donation from a pharmaceutical company, is broadly obtuse and a particularly dangerous public health decision. To do it while manufacturing the very same drug in India—where production costs are cheaper—is morally repugnant.

For Indian patients, the betrayal by their own government has been breathtaking.

The Indian health ministry agreed to the terms of donation in closed-door meetings between officials of the TB program and representatives of pharmaceutical companies Johnson & Johnson and Otsuka, the details of which are not in the public domain. The Indian government received four hundred doses of delamanid and twenty thousand doses of bedaquiline.

According to data obtained via a Right to Information request, only 4,227 patients were put on bedaquiline nationwide through all of 2018 and 2019, while the Indian government has nearly run out of its limited stock of delamanid, the *Hindu* has reported. By conservative estimates, about 150,000 people who suffer from DR TB in India are unable to take medication that is available to patients elsewhere in the world, even though one of the drugs is manufactured in their own country.

Much like those who suffered from HIV/AIDS in the early years of that disease, many Indian TB patients must grapple with a horrible reality: available drugs do not work for them, and newer medication is out of their reach.

The lack of drugs has left doctors like Udwadia to do the dirty, blood-soaked math and play God by deciding which patients receive the drug and which do not. Shreya's decision to assert her right to be treated with bedaquiline brought this human rights violation to court, even though by the time the court date arrived, she was bound to a wheelchair, weighed barely twenty-five kilograms, and could speak no more than a few sentences because she was terminally ill.

On January 20, 2017, a full five years after she was diagnosed with TB, the Delhi High Court informed Shreya's family that LRS Hospital had agreed to let Dr. Udwadia treat her with bedaquiline. The absurdly restrictive "domicile argument"—that only patients living in a five-kilometer radius of the hospitals could access medicines—did not stand the scrutiny of the court and was held to be unconstitutional.

By the time Shreya got the drugs, she had been ravaged by the disease. "She had tested negative, but there was so much delay in getting the medicines that her lungs were severely affected," Dr. Udwadia said.

"She had a miserable end."

In October 2018, she died. That year, she was one of 450,000 TB patients who died in India. She was one of the 1,400 people who died on that day in October. Activists, journalists, and lawyers who had been involved in the court case called each other the day she died. Not many, myself included, called her family. Her mother noticed.

In May 2019, I called Shreya's mother to request interviews for my book. Her mother asked me when I knew Shreya was dead.

"I heard that week."

"Why didn't you call?"

". . ."

"Where were her doctors, the activists, the journalists?"

Shreya's mother was unflinching in her condemnation: "I hope every doctor who refused her treatment suffers like me. I hope their children get tuberculosis and they have to watch them die."

She told me to never call back on that number, and the line went dead.

After the case was won, when the family returned to Patna, they faced a landlord who did not want to rent to them and friends and family members who became distant. Reporting of the trial was intrusive, brutal, and downright insensitive. Some reporters kept calling the family to check whether Shreya was dead. Her family moved houses, retreated into a shell, and hid from the glare of the Indian media.

But their anger has not receded.

Three months after Shreya's death, her treating doctors, led by Dr. Singla at LRS Hospital—who had strung her along in the court for months questioning bedaquiline's safety—published a study in the *Indian Journal of Tuberculosis*. It said they had tested bedaquiline on 290 DR TB patients and found that, by the end of six months of treatment, 98 percent of the patients had been cured.[22] "The regimen is feasible in programmatic conditions and is relatively safe," they concluded.

Six months after Shreya died, the Indian government approved bedaquiline to be made available at 150 centers across India. Every TB patient in India owes Shreya a debt that cannot be repaid.

While the Indian government was fighting one family to deny them medicines, in June 2018, South Africa became the first country to make bedaquiline part of its treatment regimen for MDR TB and XDR TB, replacing toxic injectable drugs. South Africa has 2.5 percent (fourteen thousand) of DR TB patients.

Every patient in South Africa gets bedaquiline for free.

The doctors were happier as well.

They no longer faced impossible decisions over which patients received the new drug and which didn't. "I hate having to choose which patient should get the drug and which should die. Policy makers who make this decision don't have to face the patient and deny her medicines," said Professor Jennifer Furin.

"There is no ethical, medical, or economic justification for this stand."

CHAPTER 8

———◆———

THE CURSED DUET

One of the tragic ironies of the relentless rise of TB is that there was a moment when humans had the upper hand.

In the two decades after 1940, during the great flurry of drug discoveries, people began to believe that the "war against TB" was winnable. It was thought to be on the way out, like smallpox and polio. And for a few decades after the discovery of antibiotics, cases drastically went down across the developed world. Newer, scarier diseases properly assumed greater importance.

That's when things got worse.

"We were winning the war. We believed we had the tools to control it. Globally, people were lulled into thinking of TB as a problem solved," explained Dr. Pai. "And then, everything fell apart."

The cause of the dramatic reversal in the TB story was the widespread arrival of a new and terrible affliction: HIV/AIDS.

It was unprecedented in every way, a modern plague that moved fast, quietly, and relentlessly. A poorly funded scientific community was up against a killer virus that doctors did not fully understand.

The stigma, inequity, and prejudices of mainstream society—this time against the LGBTQ community—meant the condition was neglected and allowed to snowball to pandemic proportions in just a few years.

Then scientists found out that the MO of this new, deadly killer, HIV, was to suppress your body's immunity. Immunosuppression—HIV's signature consequence—is the biggest predisposing factor for getting tuberculosis.

People living with HIV are up to twenty-one times more likely to develop TB than those without.[1] Two of the deadliest killers known to humankind worked like an efficient tag team, earning the epithet "cursed duet." "The HIV epidemic was a rude awakening. As HIV patients start succumbing to TB, suddenly there was a realization that tuberculosis was a serious problem," said Dr. Pai. The next two decades were a bloodbath as the cursed duet of infections generated a threat to human health of unparalleled proportions.

The two diseases together killed more people than World Wars I and II combined.

* * *

Few people personify righteous fury better than Larry Kramer, one of the first civilians to alert the world to the HIV epidemic. To know him is to know how it feels to be in elemental rage. According to Kramer's 1978 novel, titled *Faggots*, the origin theory of the HIV crisis was the drug-addled, orgy-filled merriment of the flower-power era.

"For Mr. Kramer, New York in the 1960s and '70s was a haven of sexual revolution, which he both participated in and later criticized," noted a certain *New York Times* profile from May 2017.[2]

During the late 1980s, as HIV cases started turning up, Kramer's novel seemed agonizingly prophetic. To his critics, he was "arrogant, self-promoting, irrationally angry and rude, cruel, deluded, double-dealing, and possibly deranged."[3] To his admirers, he was an Old Testament seer whose early warnings to the gay community about sexual profligacy and AIDS now read as eerily prescient.[4]

Larry Kramer's anger was the response of a decent man with a moral compass who saw the HIV epidemic for what it was: another vehicle for mainstream heterosexual society to oppress a homosexual minority. This was done in several insidious ways: by delaying budgets needed to fight the crisis, by denying treatment, by stigmatizing the homosexual community as being punished for their "sins."

Larry Kramer's brand of anger was a constructive response.

News about the HIV epidemic began with a small trickle of untreatable patients—five patients to be specific. In 1981, the US CDC published an article about a rare cancer in five patients from Los Angeles—all of them were gay, and all had a rare lung infection.[5] It would take another two years for the medical community to identify the culprit—the human immunodeficiency virus. In the early years of the HIV epidemic, it was known as the gay plague—the technical name for it was GRID, or gay-related immune deficiency. The formidable health challenge turned sinister when politicians and religious leaders entered the fray. American pastor and conservative thinker Reverend Jerry Falwell famously argued that "AIDS is not just God's punishment for homosexuals. It is God's punishment for the society that tolerates homosexuals."[6]

Mainstream understanding of AIDS often characterized it as a "gay disease."

AIDS quickly provided the fodder for public figures to virulently attack patients as well as the LGBTQ community. The full weight of mainstream society's morality was brought to bear upon patients and the gay community. American president Reagan did not publicly say the word "AIDS" until 1985, the fifth year of the epidemic.

Media coverage—or lack of it—only made the homophobia worse.

Articles about HIV/AIDS were often buried in the middle pages of newspapers, and respected newsrooms perpetuated flagrantly homophobic ideas. In March 1986, William F. Buckley Jr. wrote in the *New York Times* that "everyone detected with AIDS should be tattooed in the upper forearm, to protect common-needle users, and on the buttocks, to prevent the victimization of other homosexuals."[7] Panicked by the disease, Buckley offered this solution without seeing the historic parallel of etching tattoos to identify minorities. Between the science denialism of indifferent politicians, homophobia of the media, and greed of the pharmaceutical industry, the deck was stacked against HIV patients.

Around 1984, after the diagnosis of Ryan White, mainstream society had started to accept that HIV could affect straight people too.[8] Ryan White was a thirteen-year-old boy who was diagnosed with AIDS after a blood transfusion. When he returned to school, he faced AIDS-related discrimination, and his story gained national attention. Soon Ryan White became the face of public education about HIV in America, an "acceptable" face because he was a hemophiliac child—not a sexually deviant homosexual unworthy of compassion. Within a year, most Americans had become aware of AIDS and the fact that it was rapidly spreading.

Then Hollywood star Rock Hudson announced that he had AIDS in July 1985.

It was enormous news for two reasons. Not only was the disease poorly understood, but Hudson's diagnosis was also symbolic. As *TIME* pointed out when the news broke, he had "represented the old-fashioned American virtues" of the 1950s. Hudson died less than three months later, at the age of fifty-nine. The *TIME* obituary described him as "the most celebrated known victim of AIDS" who "in the last weeks of his life . . . became perhaps the most famous homosexual in the world."[9] Once heterosexual politicians realized the virus did not target minorities exclusively, Congress approved a vast increase in funding for AIDS research.

"From his misfortune good fortune may have sprung," the *TIME* obituary concluded.

In the 1990s, AIDS research made serious progress, and celebrities were an important factor in maintaining the momentum of the search for a cure. In November 1991, thirty-two-year-old LA Lakers point guard Magic Johnson revealed in a press conference that he was HIV positive and would be retiring from basketball. "I will now become a spokesman for the HIV virus, and I want young people to know that they can practice safe sex," he said.[10] Two weeks after Johnson's announcement, another celebrity came out with the heartbreaking diagnosis: the lead singer of Queen, Freddie Mercury. He died of complications from AIDS-related pneumonia on November 24, 1991, at the age of forty-five. About seventy-two thousand people attended a benefit concert held at London's Wembley Stadium, raising millions for AIDS research.

In 1987, Larry Kramer cofounded the group ACT UP (the AIDS Coalition to Unleash Power), and the members organized themselves into a sophisticated protest movement. In the decades since, no public health movement has been able to come anywhere near what "ACT UPpers" managed to do.

ACT UP came into being when Kramer made a speech in which he asked two-thirds of his audience to stand up, whereupon he told them they would be dead in five years.[11] "If what you are hearing doesn't rouse you to anger, fury, rage, and action, gay men will have no future here on earth."

Few movements have used nonviolent protests as effectively as ACT UPpers.

Kramer tapped into the anger that had brought patients together. ACT UP's original goal was to demand the release of experimental AIDS drugs, and they put considerable pressure on pharmaceutical companies to cut the prices for them.

The New York chapter of ACT UP routinely drew more than eight hundred people to its weekly meetings and thus became the largest and most influential of all the American chapters.

By early 1988, ACT UP had active chapters in Los Angeles, Boston, Chicago, and San Francisco. By the beginning of 1990, ACT UP had spread throughout the United States and around the globe, with more than one hundred chapters worldwide.

For the next decade, ACT UP was the standard-bearer for protesting governmental and societal indifference to the AIDS epidemic. The US government was trying to keep the community from panicking, whereas ACT UPpers insisted there was every reason to panic—and, in fact, panic was entirely necessary.

In October 1988, ACT UP organized its most success-ful demonstrations when it shut down the Food and Drug

Administration (FDA) for a day.[12] Around fifteen hundred people stood outside the FDA, hoisting a black banner that read "Federal Death Administration." All day, they chanted the rehashed anti-Vietnam war chant, "Hey, hey, FDA, how many people have you killed today?" When the police were called in, the officers, afraid to touch people from the HIV community, were wearing surgical gloves.

A month later, on September 14, 1989, seven ACT UP members infiltrated the New York Stock Exchange wearing suits and fake trader ID badges, carrying chains, handcuffs, and foghorns.[13] The traders were stunned, and some began shouting from the balconies, "Die, faggots!" and "Mace them!" ACT UPpers chained themselves to protest the high price of the only FDA-approved AIDS drug, AZT. Pharmaceutical company Burroughs-Wellcome owned the drug and had originally priced it at $10,000 for a year's dosage. It lowered the price to $8,000 when threatened with a congressional inquiry.

AZT, at that point, was the most expensive drug ever sold.[14] Within weeks of the stock exchange protest, Burroughs-Wellcome reduced the price of AZT by 20 percent, to $6,400 a year, claiming that it had been planning to do so all along. Then the protestors upped the ante.

Their next target was organized religion and media. About three months after the stock exchange event, in December 1989, around forty-five hundred activists gathered for the Stop the Church campaign outside St. Patrick Cathedral in New York. Dozens entered the cathedral, interrupted mass, chanted slogans, or lay down in the aisles. One protestor broke a communion wafer and threw it to the floor. One hundred and eleven were arrested.[15] ACT UP had targeted the Catholic Church because New York's cardinal was a homophobe. Cardinal John O'Connor had been using his influence in New York City to keep the Board of Education away from teaching safe sex practices and distributing condoms. From the church ACT UP moved on to the national media. They organized a Day of Desperation, when activists entered the studio of the *CBS Evening News* and shouted, "AIDS is news!"[16] The next day, activists displayed two banners in the iconic ticket hall of Grand Central Station. One said, "Money for AIDS, Not for War," and another said, "One AIDS Death Every 8 Minutes." One of the banners was attached to bundles of balloons that lifted it up to the station's celestial ceiling.

Through it all was the animating, angry, divisive, but never absent figure of Larry Kramer. "I was known as the angriest man in the world, mainly because I discovered that anger got you further than being nice. And when we started to break through in the media, I was better TV than someone who was nice," he told the *New York Times* reporter.[17] HIV activists of the 1980s needed to rely on theater because that's what underdogs do. Because American patients found leaders like Larry Kramer to organize, educate, and agitate, eventually mainstream society, through instruments like courts, media, and public tolerance, adapted to the reality of the epidemic.

Science delivered too.

The speed of research, treatment, and public health education, while tragically slow, eventually picked up pace. Within a few years, HIV treatments had advanced enough for Magic Johnson to return to basketball. In January 1996, he signed a $2.5 million contract for the second half of the season. While the American narrative of the HIV movement is a classic David versus Goliath story, in which David eventually prevailed, that was not the story everywhere.

In Africa and Asia, David never stood a chance.

Even though there were famous deaths from AIDS, the epidemic unfolded in the developing world without much to stop it. To this day, what was happening in the 1980s in America continues to happen in low- and middle-income countries around the world, where patients are brown and black. AIDS has, however, fallen out of the headlines.

The cursed duet is now at its deadliest.

PART III

CHAPTER 9

———◆———

WRETCHED OF THE EARTH

When you have HIV, you don't *die* of HIV. This virus's MO is to create an opportunity for *other diseases* to plunder the infected body—these ailments are called "opportunistic infections."

HIV switches off the body's immune system, and tuberculosis ravages it.

Tuberculosis is the leading opportunistic infection among HIV patients and, globally, the most common, immediate cause of death among HIV patients. Both TB (bacteria) and HIV (virus) are master mutators. They have lengthy periods of latency, where they lie low and wait for immunity to come down.

Neither disease kills its host immediately, which is a huge evolutionary advantage that allows the disease to spread. Once infected, the patient can remain asymptomatic, sometimes for decades, while the virus continues to multiply internally.

By 1999, TB was responsible for 30 percent of the 2.8 million deaths in HIV patients globally.[1] As of 2020, one-third of the 40 million people living with HIV were infected with TB, and 90 percent of them die within months of contracting TB without proper treatment.[2]

In 2021, TB continues to be the leading cause of death among HIV-infected people. As per WHO's Global TB Report (2020), out of the ten million cases of TB worldwide, an estimated 8.2 percent were coinfected with HIV.[3]

While both diseases are under control in the developed world, they are not in the developing world. Most developing and under-developed nations could not cope with the HIV outbreak. Historical pillaging, and the ravages of colonialism that endured for years after the colonizers, left these nations with insufficient hospitals, infrastructure, and able governments. In India, which was under British rule until 1947, there was additional colonial baggage: laws passed by the empire that made homosexuality a crime.

The land of the *Kama Sutra* succumbed to Victorian values.

In the colonized world, homosexual communities were driven underground, making it more challenging for them to organize, agitate, and educate. Patients were, understandably, scared to seek treatment because they were treated like criminals. One arm of the Indian government, the health ministry, asked them to come forward for treatment, while another arm, the police, arrested them when they did.

Patients chose to live with the disease, condemning themselves and those around them to a brutal life and an equally brutal death.

Two regions were most affected: sub-Saharan Africa, where 63 percent of all AIDS-related deaths have occurred, and Asia, where the largest percentage of the human population infected by TB lives. Patients living in these regions fought big pharmaceutical companies hard for years before they got access to HIV medicines. In the early 1990s, first-generation anti-HIV drugs cost $10,000–$15,000 per year, per patient.

In Uganda, Dr. Peter Mugyenyi was among the doctors diagnosing HIV patients, giving them the bad news, and sending them home to die. Most patients in Uganda, and in sub-Saharan Africa, could not afford AZT, the first drug to be approved by the US FDA in 1987.

On July 9, 2000, Dr. Mugyenyi appeared at the International HIV Conference in Durban and asked a blunt question, which became famous in public health circles: "Where are the drugs?"

Dr. Mugyenyi's answer was even more forthright: "The drugs are where the disease is not. And where is the disease? The disease is where the drugs are not."

Pharmaceutical companies have always made the majority of their profits in Western countries, or "commercially viable" markets. By 2020, the revenue of the global pharmaceutical market was US$1.27 trillion, of which the North American market share was 48.7 percent. The EU has a 14 percent share.[4] African nations, which were suffering the worst of the HIV epidemic, accounted for 0.7 percent of the global pharmaceutical market. Despite being the worst affected, the African continent remained on the sidelines during the first two decades of the HIV response.

As a result, AIDS became an entirely different beast there. By the 1990s, different regions of the world were showing different patterns of spread of HIV/AIDS.

In Africa, HIV patients were eleven times more likely to die within five years and more than one hundred times more likely to develop Kaposi's sarcoma, a cancer linked to yet another virus.[5] By the time Dr. Mugyenyi made the speech at the Durban conference, the worst of the epidemic was over for Americans, but it was roaring like a fireball across southern Africa.

In sub-Saharan Africa, more than twenty-five million people were infected with HIV, and more than seventeen million had already died. South Africa, a country the size of Texas and carrying heavy colonial baggage, had been brought to its knees by this epidemic. Dr. Mugyenyi's book *Genocide by Denial: How Profiteering from HIV/AIDS Killed Millions* documents the AIDS epidemic from an African perspective.[6] The US government, a rich and wealthy nation, closed its eyes and turned away, until the 2003 State of the Union address in which President Bush announced PEPFAR (President's Emergency Plan for AIDS Relief), the single largest commitment toward the HIV/AIDS crisis.

In September 2000, the European Commission in Brussels invited health ministers, heads of government, and chief executives of major pharmaceutical companies for high-level talks. Professor Furin cited this meeting as a comparable example of scientific racism toward black and brown patients. The European Commission, WHO, and the Joint United Nations Programme on HIV/AIDS had come together to discuss the issue of access to HIV medicines in the developing world.[7] There was a "debate" within the public health community about giving African nations access to newly discovered HIV medicines, in which some dismissively racist voices were raised: Jan Raaijmakers, director of science and business development at pharmaceutical company GlaxoSmithKline, which owned the patent for AZT, said of the Africans begging for the drug, "They are mostly illiterates. Can't read the information on the leaflets in the drug packets and have to cope without a healthcare system that can tell them about the disease they have."

Not having a robust health-care system was the reason to deny health care altogether.

Andrew Natsios, head of foreign disaster assistance at USAID from 1989 to 1991, chimed in: "The biggest problem for antiretrovirals—this sounds small and some people, if you've traveled to rural Africa, you know this; this is not a criticism, just a different world—people do not know what watches and clocks are. They do not use Western means for telling the time; they use the sun."

In this way, a steady stream of racist tropes denied African patients the medicines.

Twenty-four million Africans were dying from AIDS by 2000, and there were protests across African nations to access affordable HIV medicines. By conservative estimates, ten million people died in Africa during the delay in getting AZT to Africa.

In South Africa, the country's problems were compounded by an HIV denialist government.

In 1999, Thabo Mbeki succeeded Nelson Mandela as South Africa's president. Even as the country's neighbors ramped up prevention and treatment efforts, Mbeki—president from 1999 until he resigned under pressure in September 2008—publicly challenged the scientific consensus that HIV causes AIDS. His health minister, Manto Tshabalala-Msimang, promoted herbal remedies, including beetroot, garlic, and lemon, as alternatives for antiretrovirals. It was a terrible, unforgivable throwback to the prescientific folk remedies of 150 years past.

In 2009, a Harvard study calculated the full extent of science denialism.[8] More than 330,000 people died prematurely from HIV/AIDS between 2000 and 2005 due to the Mbeki government's obstruction of lifesaving treatment.[9]

In 2005, at the peak of the HIV epidemic, there were about nine hundred deaths a day. It was the reason why South Africa had one of the severest HIV/AIDS epidemics in the world—and in turn a severe TB epidemic, second only to India. In July 2000, the pharmaceutical company Boehringer Ingelheim offered to donate its HIV drug nevirapine, which could prevent the transmission of HIV from mother to child, during labor. But South Africa restricted the availability of nevirapine to two pilot sites per province until December 2002 (much like access to bedaquiline was limited to six sites in India). The same Harvard study concluded that around thirty-five thousand HIV-infected babies were born who could have been protected from the virus.

Horrified by the Mbeki denialism, the international scientific community signed the Durban Declaration, a petition that endorsed the mainstream scientific view that HIV did indeed cause AIDS.

As late as summer 2006, South Africa's health minister, Tshabalala-Msimang, astonished participants at an international AIDS conference in Toronto by presenting a government public-health display that focused on beetroot, olive oil, garlic, lemons, and African potatoes. This stance earned her the derisive nicknames Dr. Garlic and Dr. Beetroot from critics. Antiretroviral drugs were included in the display only after furious protests.[10] The Mbeki era also fostered a profound mistrust of scientific medicine, the consequences of which also cannot be quantified. Mbeki eventually relented, and antiretrovirals become available via the public health system in 2004. It owed more to legal intervention than to a change in Mbeki's personal beliefs on the matter; in 2002, South Africa's highest court ruled that the government must make the medicines available.

Mbeki, an economist and one of Africa's most respected leaders, has never disavowed the view that HIV medicines are Western inventions aimed at maiming Africans. Mbeki has been notoriously unwilling to speak about the era of his AIDS denialism.

He has never apologized for what happened under his leadership in South Africa, and the consequences are generational: 7.5 million living with HIV as of 2019, and 5.2 million on antiretroviral therapy.

In 2019, South Africa was home to 36 percent of the global total 38 million HIV patients, 11 percent of 1.7 million new infections, and 10 percent of 690,000 AIDS-related deaths.[11]

The second-largest program was India's, which was treating 747,175 people at the time.[12] India implemented a progressive HIV policy, impressively containing the epidemic through its national AIDS program. The country's HIV program—which had a vocal community and activist base—was one of its best-performing health initiatives.

It would not last.

While South Africa's science denialism was in the past by 2021, in India it had reared its head, sponsored by a ruling party that says cow urine can treat cancer. Under Modi's leadership, India has invested heavily in pseudoscience. Soon after coming to power in 2014, the Modi administration cut budgets to flagship health programs, including those for HIV/AIDS and tuberculosis interventions.

The impact was immediate.

The supply of antiretroviral drugs, which had been erratic since December 2013, worsened. Stocks depleted throughout 2014, until in January 2015 the shelves were empty. For nearly nine excruciating months, every antiretroviral therapy center in the country had run out of at least one drug for several weeks.[13]

The next blow to India's HIV program came in April 2016, when the Modi administration fired the bulk of HIV experts—who had been funded by international donor organizations and consulting with the health ministry—en masse. Ninety consultants, nearly one-fourth, were asked to leave at the end of June 2016.[14] The experts were fired for being "foreign funded" as the Modi administration clamped down on the influence of international agencies and NGOs on public policy in India. It was a deadly blow to a staggering HIV program, and the program has never recovered from it.

In 2016, the annual HIV conference returned to Durban—sixteen years after the Mbeki era. The mood was upbeat, and the conversations among the attendees were relaxed; words like "elimination" were thrown around. Such words risk making us dangerously complacent.

Thirty-eight million people currently live with AIDS, a disease that claimed the lives of nearly 690,000 people in 2019. Experts predict that by 2030, 100 million people will have been infected with HIV. Complacency about HIV/AIDS and reduced funding risk advances toward ending the global epidemic.

Of the thirty-eight million infected with HIV, only twenty-two million have access to treatment.

"Too many people don't get care," the World Health Organization's chief, Tedros Adhanom Ghebreyesus, told the AIDS 2018 conference. "We will not meet our targets," he warned.[15]

* * *

On February 6, 2001, Cipla Pharmaceuticals offered the triple antiretroviral cocktail—the gold standard of HIV treatment—for $350 per patient per year.

Overnight, the price for HIV treatment fell from $15,000 per patient per year to a dollar a day, deliberately priced to be below the symbolic threshold. It was a watershed moment. The *New York Times* made it front-page news.

Cipla had been founded for this very reason. In 1939, when Mahatma Gandhi called for a boycott of all British products, including medicines, he visited Cipla and motivated the founder to make essential medicines for the country.

During World War II, when India faced shortage a of life-saving drugs, Cipla manufactured them as its duty to the nation.

In the documentary *Fire in the Blood*, *New York Times* health reporter Donald McNeil, who was tracking the story of HIV drug prices, said Cipla's pricing was "the dam breaking."[16]

India, and its nascent pharmaceutical industry, basked in the glory. Dr. Yusuf Hamied, Cipla's charming director, was at the center of it all.

On September 20, 2000, at the same European Commission conference in Brussels where Raaijmakers and Natsios were arguing against sending drugs to Africa because Africans could not tell time, Dr. Hamied made a different proposal.[17] He stared at an unfriendly audience of pharmaceutical multinationals and mostly white European leaders and said, "Friends, I represent the needs and aspirations of the third world."[18]

He proceeded to make three offers: he'd sell his HIV cocktail at $800 per year (and offered a further discounted rate of $600 to government on bulk procurement); transfer technology to African governments willing to manufacture their own medicines; and throw in nevirapine, the drug that limited mother-to-child transmission, for free. He closed his speech saying, "We call upon the participants of this conference to do what their conscience dictates."

"You could hear the breath being sucked out of the room," said Bill Haddad, former *New York Post* investigative journalist and generic drug manufacturer.[19]

Not a single government or global health organization took him up on his offer. Shocked by the refusal, Dr. Hamied still manage to disrupt the monopoly. He single-handedly broke the cartel of the big drug companies by offering to supply AIDS drugs at less than a tenth of their prices to Médecins Sans Frontières, which did accept it.

GlaxoSmithKline's former CEO Jean-Pierre Garnier called Cipla and Dr. Hamied "pirates."[20] To Indian doctors and patients, he was the Robin Hood of drugs. What his eighty-year-old pharma company did proved to be the turning point in the history of HIV/AIDS. The pirate had developed a revolutionary three-drug anti-HIV cocktail—nevirapine, didanosine, and zidovudine—and offered it to the developing nations at one-thirtieth of what Big Pharma was charging.

Blindsided, Big Pharma had to lower prices to match Cipla at less than a dollar a day. Today, one in three people living with HIV in the world takes a Cipla drug for treatment. This pharmaceutical coup was possible because of a brilliant legal reading of patent law.

India, a young, ambitious, and proud nation, had a patent law that placed patients before profits.

In 1972, Prime Minister Indira Gandhi had modified the Raj-era copyright and patent law of 1911. With the amendments, the new nation recognized only "process patents." On April 20, 1972, the Indian government decided that in food and health, companies could not patent a product; they could only patent a *process*. Because of this interpretation of law, it became possible to produce and sell patented drugs as long as they were manufactured through unique processes.[21]

In an address to the WHO in 1981, Mrs. Gandhi had said that "no one will be allowed to make profit out of illness and misery of the poor people in India." Dr. Hamied could reverse engineer HIV medicines and sell them for a dollar a day in 2001 because of the Indian Patent Law of 1972.

Good-quality, affordable Indian-made generic drugs changed the course of the HIV epidemic by taking the drugs to where the disease was: Africa. By the time Cipla's drugs arrived, 24.5 million people were living with HIV in Africa—and only one in a thousand had access to medicines.[22]

James Packard Love, director of Knowledge Ecology International, a Washington, DC–based nongovernmental organization, had been investigating Big Pharma's drug price policies for years. He was investigating *why* HIV drugs cost as much as they did.

In *Fire in the Blood*, he said,

You know, if it was the lives of white people at stake, how could the international community not know what it cost to save lives? Why did I have to be the person to go out and figure out what it costs to make an AIDS drug? I didn't work for the government, I didn't work for the World Health Organization, or UNAIDS or the CIA, or anyone else. I just worked for this little NGO. What was really going on is the WHO didn't want to know what it cost to make an AIDS cocktail. UNAIDS didn't want to know what it cost to make an AIDS cocktail. The United States government didn't want to know what it cost to make an AIDS cocktail. And why didn't they want to know? Because if the public understood that you can make an AIDS cocktail for $200 to $300, it wouldn't look very good. It would be an absolute intolerable set of facts to have out there. So the way they were trying to manage the situation was to deliberately stay as ignorant and as stupid as possible about what the facts were. It was just a really deep form of racism, I thought. It was just a completely morally repugnant situation.[23]

Multinational pharmaceutical companies—Boehringer Ingelheim, GlaxoSmithKline, Bristol-Meyers Squib, Hoffman-LaRoche, and Merck—all with patents on antiretrovirals, were not letting this happen without a fight.[24]

When drugs became affordable for African nations, pharmaceutical companies used patent laws to keep them from getting to Africa. The patent hurdles restricted bulk procurement by agencies such as UNICEF, the International Dispensary Association, and Médecins Sans Frontières, who were procuring drugs from India and distributing in Africa.

They did this by an aggressive two-pronged use of patent law: block production of generics and block exports and imports. This badly reasoned approach—especially from a public health point of view—resulted in a false shortage, which then created a situation in which drugs had to be rationed.

As a result, doctors had to decide which patients lived and which ones died based on factors such as how many children would be orphaned, which patient was too ill, and other unquantifiable criteria. The ethical contortions were grating to Dr. Peter Mugyenyi, head of one of the biggest HIV response centers in Africa, the JCRC or Joint Clinical Research Centre.

He was watching patients die at his clinic in Uganda and could overhear dying patients matter-of-factly discussing their decision to kill their AIDS-infected loved ones as an act of mercy, to save them the slow, miserable, lonely decline.

On many days, Dr. Mugyenyi was left with wailing orphans as both parents succumbed to HIV. In his book *Genocide by Denial*, he writes, "There was no escape. The problem had either to be endured or addressed. If this was not justification enough to take the bull by its horns, then I do not know a better one."

Without consulting his government, Dr. Mugyenyi contacted Cipla in India to ask if they would supply his center, JCRC, with antiretroviral drugs. It was reckless bravado by any measure. Dr. Mugyenyi had tossed a hot potato at Cipla, which was in enough trouble already. The five pharmaceutical companies with patents on HIV drugs, including GlaxoSmithKline, had accused Dr. Hamied of patent infringements when he announced his cocktail. He knew processing Dr. Mugyenyi's order would only make matters worse.

Cipla wrote back asking for legal guarantees and was assured that when (not if) law enforcement knocked at the door, it would be Dr. Mugyenyi's problem and not Cipla's. With that, Dr. Hamied agreed to fulfill the order.

As soon as the medicines arrived, they were impounded by customs officials at Entebbe Airport, and Dr. Mugyenyi was placed under arrest for importation of unauthorized drugs. The decision to import HIV drugs had brought things to a head, exactly as Dr. Mugyenyi had hoped.

As the first major international public health emergency in an era of newly minted patent laws, the HIV epidemic exposed fault lines in trade policies that had serious racial implications. It was hard to ignore that the patent holders were largely in the developed world while patients were in the colonized world.

Initially, the full force of the law was brought to bear upon Dr. Mugyenyi. The Ugandan government decided to return the medicines at Dr. Mugyenyi's expense. But there was no doubt who occupied the moral high ground: the epidemic was out of control, a batch of lifesaving drugs were stuck at Entebbe Airport, and the doctor who was trying to save his patients had been arrested. As journalists and activists started working the phones, politicians were suddenly made conscious of the optics of it all.

The Ugandan president, Yoweri Museveni, called a crisis meeting.

Dr. Mugyenyi did not deny the charges leveled against him. At the meeting, he explained his decision calmly: "I did not try to smuggle the drugs but presented them to legal official channels for clearance. What remains is for you to take a decision to allow them in or not."

He did not have to struggle to convince the Ugandan government to do the right thing. HIV was raging across the country; many politicians had relatives or friends who had tested positive. The Ugandan government asked its lawyers to look for loopholes to get the drugs in. The focus of this crisis meeting quickly changed from determining whether to throw Dr. Mugyenyi in jail to finding a way to get the medicines to patients.

The lawyers found a loophole.

As in the US, the Ugandan national laws had provision for an emergency clause; it allowed the government to clear the drugs in the interest of national health.

Once the solution was found, people turned to Dr. Mugyenyi, telling him this would be his "reprieve." That's when he threw the gauntlet down, saying, "I'm sorry; I cannot accept this offer to let the drugs in." He explained to his stunned audience, a roomful of lawyers, bureaucrats, and politicians, that one consignment of drugs might postpone a few deaths but that AIDS was a lifelong illness. Any decision that did not guarantee sustained access to antiretrovirals was a half measure. In a historic decision, the lawyers argued the same emergency clause could be used for subsequent consignments.

For the first time since the beginning of the HIV epidemic, universal access to medicines was an achievable dream.

As soon as the drugs were released from Entebbe Airport, two quick decisions were made. Both would turn that day into the "best of [Dr. Mugyenyi's] AIDS career."[25] First, the number of patients on antiretrovirals drastically increased, and a second, even bigger order for drugs was immediately placed. Two representatives of large pharmaceutical companies—which Dr. Mugyenyi has never named—approached him and offered to match Cipla's price. Ever the trickster, Dr. Mugyenyi called Cipla the minute the pharma reps left his office and told them he did not need to import drugs, as the brand-name ones were available to him at the same price. Cipla offered to lower the price further.

From that day on, the cost of common first-line AIDS drugs was never the same.

A competition between Indian generics and Big Pharma drug manufacturers had begun in earnest.

Dr. Mugyenyi had made the West listen to the needs of the developing world by using market forces against their monopolies and by shaming their indifference—"until the stink of it all reached them in the bastions of their privileged circumstances, far away from the wretched of the earth."

CHAPTER 10

PATENTS VERSUS PATIENTS

The World Trade Organization (WTO) is the centerpiece of the global system of rules, institutions, and beliefs dictating the ownership and flow of knowledge, science, technology, and every other intangible intellectual asset.

It is to global trade what WHO is to global health: the nerve center of how knowledge, and by extension wealth, flows. Intellectual property (IP) laws and trade between nations is the most lucrative and jargon-dense vertical of WTO's functions.

Its flagship policy, among the least examined from the point of view of the developing world, is the TRIPS Agreement (the Agreement on Trade-Related Aspects of Intellectual Property Rights).

It was enforced in 1995 and is the single most important accord on IP of the twentieth century. It establishes minimum global standards to protect new ideas, especially and not coincidentally those from pharmaceutical companies.

The WTO is heavily influenced by the American government. It services oligopolies while offering a series of condescending aid policies and donation programs, run by the rich but aimed at serving the status quo.

The donation programs of pharmaceutical companies, much like aid from developed nations, has created a vicious cycle of allowing false generosity. In his book *Pedagogy of the Oppressed*, twentieth-century Brazilian educator Paulo Freire defines "false generosity" as follows: "In order to have the continued opportunity to express their 'generosity,' the oppressor must perpetuate injustice as well. An unjust social order is the permanent fount of this 'generosity,' which is nourished by death, despair, and poverty. This is why dispensers of false generosity become desperate at the slightest threat to its source."

To developing nations, one example of false generosity is the Gates Foundation.

To understand health, one must begin with technology. Drugs, vaccines, and testing kits are all technology. And everything is someone's intellectual property, or so we have been led to believe.

The fount of global health inequities flows from how technology is transferred and on whose terms.

In November 2020, the *New York Times* quoted Amir Attaran, professor of law and medicine at the University of Ottawa, who said, "The Gates Foundation presence has been, at best, an adjunct to W.H.O. and at worst a hostile takeover and a usurpation."[1] The Gates Foundation is the largest private donor to the WHO. Officials from the agency—which receives millions of dollars from the foundation—make decisions behind closed doors, peppered with clashes of interest, good intentions, and huge blind spots.

At the heart of it all is Bill Gates, one of the world's richest men—not a scientist, not a doctor, and not an elected official.

Gates has emerged as the world's de facto public health leader after having spent the post-HIV decades defending monopoly medicine. In April 2021, the *New Republic* published an essay on Bill Gates titled "Vaccine Monster."[2] In it, journalist Alexander Zaitchik wrote, "Bill Gates's position on intellectual property was consistent with a lifelong ideological commitment to knowledge monopolies, forged during a vengeful teenage crusade against the open-source programming culture of the 1970s. As it happens, a novel use of one category of intellectual property—copyright, applied to computer code—made Gates the richest man in the world for most of two decades beginning in 1995."

As his company morphed into a giant, Gates started expanding his influence in global health. In a November 2020 profile in the *New York Times*, Professor Manjari Mahajan, who teaches global health and philanthrocapitalism at the New School, said Gates brought a "technocratic expertise and power rather than a discourse of human rights and activism."[3]

The Gates Foundation employs former pharmaceutical executives in its top ranks, including Dr. Trevor Mundel, who had been the global head of development at Novartis, and Emilio Emini, previously a senior vice president of vaccine research at Pfizer. Gates became interested in immunizations in the late 1990s, when Microsoft was facing an antitrust case. He declared war on Netscape, attempting to smother it by bundling Microsoft's own free Internet Explorer browser with Windows and pressuring other companies to use it instead of Netscape Navigator.

Gates has the mind of a genius and the morals of a thug, as was evident with Netscape's abrupt end.

He often descends from Mount Olympus to get into fist fights with small companies like Netscape. As Netscape struggled to stay afloat, the US government sued Gates for anticompetitive behavior. By the late 1990s, Microsoft had been having skirmishes with the Department of Justice and the Federal Trade Commission for almost a decade. In 1998, Gates testified in front of Congress in rousing defense of monopolies. The internet was threatening to make his operating systems obsolete.

Netscape Navigator, more popular than Windows Explorer, had to be cut down. Microsoft savagely drove Netscape out of business. It pressured companies not to work with Netscape and started giving away its own browser, Internet Explorer, for free.

Gates, champion of new ideas, has no qualms killing them if they are not his.

He is not the first one with that flaw; he is just the tip of an iceberg that formed over centuries. The implicit assumption—of knowledge as a monopoly—can be traced all the way back to the colonial era.

The idea that ideas belong to singular individuals, and must be protected, stems from an unsettling view of the developing world. It is buttressed by the West's view of itself as an ideal system, one for the Global South to emulate.

In Africa, Asia, and the Pacific, the formal introduction of IP laws began in the late nineteenth century with a single purpose: to enrich European colonial powers.

The first IP treaty was the Paris Convention for the Protection of Industrial Property, signed in Paris on March 20, 1883, as the scramble for Africa was heating up. Within a year, Otto von Bismarck, the first chancellor of Germany, organized the Berlin Conference. Its chief purpose, in 1884, was to regulate trade in Africa, and the colonizers moved swiftly to impose new laws, authorities, and institutions throughout their territories.

The colonies were not at the negotiating table.

In 1893, the secretariats of the Berne and Paris Conventions were merged to form the United International Bureaux for Protection of Intellectual Property, the predecessor of the World Intellectual Property Organization (WIPO)—neither name arrived at with placards in mind.

The two conventions—Berlin and Paris—ushered in a period of concentrated plunder of wealth from colonies, eliminating or overriding autonomy and self-governance in the colonies. With these laws, France and Great Britain laid the foundations for an enduring influence on the legal framework in Africa and Asia. The two conventions would also mark the beginning of long-standing tensions between the Global North and the South, setting us on the winding, rocky, political road that would culminate in the TRIPS Agreement.

India, the crown jewel of the British Empire, acquired a patent law in 1856—long before many European countries. By 1911, Britain had added a copyright act throughout its empire, including in East Africa, Malaysia, and Nigeria.

The colonialists may have wanted to convince themselves that they were on a "civilizing mission," but from the start the British East India Company was a profit-driven enterprise. Even though the British came to India to look for silk, spices, and other goods, they were quick to see the benefit of blocking India's industrial development. A nation that had been known for making textiles, steel, and ships was reduced to a raw-material-producing colony.

The looting began, predictably, with unequal trade agreements that focused on extraction of resources through the nineteenth century. The free trade policy of the empire ruined India's artisans and enabled Britain to build a world-leading textile industry. Further, the primary education of Indians was neglected.

Shashi Tharoor's book *Inglorious Empire: What the British Did to India* notes that India's literacy rate at independence in 1947 was a mere 16 percent (8 percent for women). Moreover, some seventeen million Indians died of hunger in the years 1891 to 1900. In 1943, the Bengal famine killed another four million people.

Mountains and statesmen are better viewed from a distance. From India, where millions of Indians died as wars raged in Europe, Winston Churchill looks like nothing else but a brutal bully and a racist.

In the bleak days of May and June 1940, Britain's new prime minister was a desperate man. As the head of a nation that had made territorial grabs one after another, getting away with it each time, Churchill was now in an unfamiliar position: begging for American aid in a war that was going Hitler's way.

Within a year, France had fallen. The German war machine had engulfed Czechoslovakia, Hungary, Austria, Denmark, the Netherlands, Belgium, and Norway and was set to invade Great Britain. For the first two years, America refused to get involved in the European war. Churchill's wartime speeches, made between 1940 and 1941, were aimed as much at raising morale among the British people as they were at persuading Americans, especially Roosevelt, to support the Allied war effort.

The speeches—filled with language of moral high ground about fighting the tyranny and barbarism of Nazis—never acknowledged what he, his government, and his empire had done to the colonies as either tyranny or barbarism. When Churchill famously said, "I have nothing to offer but blood, toil, tears, and sweat," he omitted to mention that also on offer were Indian bodies, blood, toil, tears, and sweat.

All the while, he refused to give up the crown's favorite colony, India. In British India, signs of "Indians and dogs not allowed" were common at clubs and in public spaces, in line with the racial etiquette of the Jim Crow South or apartheid South Africa. During the Bengal famine, Churchill blamed the victims, arguing that the suffering resulted from "breeding like rabbits," when in truth, Bengal was starving because Allied soldiers were being fed by India's paddy.

Churchill, even today eulogized as a great statesman, was a genuine racist who hated Asians for their "slit eyes and pig tails."[4] To him, people from India were "the beastliest people in the world next to the Germans."[5] He admitted that he "did not really think that black people were as capable or as efficient as white people."[6]

As the war drew to a bloody end and Allied powers negotiated victory over their enemies, American president Franklin D. Roosevelt was instrumental in calling out the empire's hypocrisy in keeping its colonies in a stranglehold while calling Nazis evil for the same thing.

As recounted in the book *As He Saw It*, by Roosevelt's son Elliot, Roosevelt laid it all on the table for Churchill:

> Father broke in. "Yes. Those Empire trade agreements are a case in point. It's because of them that the people of India and Africa, of all the colonial Near East and Far East, are still as backward as they are." . . .
>
> "You mentioned India," he [Churchill] growled.
>
> "Yes. I can't believe that we can fight a war against fascist slavery, and at the same time not work to free people all over the world from a backward colonial policy."
>
> Churchill's neck reddened and he crouched forward. "Mr. President, England does not propose for a moment to lose its favored

position among the British Dominions. The trade that has made England great shall continue, and under conditions prescribed by England's ministers."

"You see," said Father slowly, "it is along in here somewhere that there is likely to be some disagreement between you, Winston, and me."[7]

In 2003, Angus Maddison, a British economist, calculated that India's share of the global GDP went from 24.4 percent to 4.2 percent during two and a half centuries of colonial rule. In 1884, the British state had a total income of 203 million pounds, of which more than half came from its overseas territories, including 74 million pounds from India. "Loot," the Urdu/Hindi word for plunder, was one of the first Indian words to enter the English language. Economist Utsa Patnaik asserts that "between 1765 and 1938, the drain amounted to £9.2 trillion ($45 trillion)."[8]

To enable this plunder, Britain built India's vast railway network—much the same way thieves have getaway cars to move the loot quickly. France did the same.

In every colony, IP laws loaded the dice in favor of the empire. The TRIPS Agreement is the legal inheritor of the long shadow of colonization, and philathrocapitalist billionaires like Bill Gates, who got rich on knowledge monopolies, are the tip of this iceberg.

The second phase of radical change in IP laws came during the postwar era of decolonization (1940s–1960s). Newly independent nations wanted to favor local producers, protect local markets, funnel investment into new sectors, and regulate foreign trade. This sparked efforts to substantially revise their IP laws. But most newly independent countries maintained strong political, legal, and financial links with former colonizers; they had to because they had emerged from the colonial era with weak infrastructure and fragile governments.

So, they remained within the framework of copyright laws enacted by the British.

It took India a quarter century to revise the legal strictures. A year after independence, India set up the Patent Enquiry Committee (1948–1950). This farsighted committee concluded that "the Indian patent system has failed in its main purpose, namely, to stimulate inventions among Indians and to encourage the development and exploitation of new inventions for industrial purposes in the country so as to secure the benefits thereof to the largest section of the public."[9] Based on this committee's advice, India amended the 1911 Patents and Design Act, tailoring the law to national priorities. The country needed to increase access to medicines at lower prices, prioritize industrial capacity building, and foster R&D in areas of national significance and rural development.

The strongest reform did not arrive until 1970, when India adopted the new patent law. It allowed innovators to patent methods or processes related to new medicines *but not the medicines themselves*. The new law also limited the term of patents in areas of social concern, such as food and health, to seven years (in contrast to fourteen years for other inventions).

This law became the legal foundation for India's generic drug industry that made it the pharmacy of the developing world.

Brazil, Mexico, and Argentina similarly lowered standards of patent protection to stimulate local production of generic medicines. The reformist IP agenda of postcolonial nations was not welcomed, especially by pharmaceutical oligopolies of the developed countries who had hitherto dominated the international market for medicines.

This growing activism provoked concern within the developed world, which, partly in response, established the WIPO in 1967. It would act as a brake on the progress of the developing world.

In her book *The Implementation Game: The TRIPS Agreement and the Global Politics of Intellectual Property Reform in Developing Countries*, Carolyn Deere notes that "eighty per cent of patents granted worldwide at that time were owned by major corporations from five industrialized countries. Further, over 80 per cent of the patents in force in developing countries were held by foreigners and registered on the basis of research conducted elsewhere. Developing countries thus argued that international patent rules were intrinsically unbalanced in favour of developed countries."[10]

By the 1970s, developing countries held only around 1 percent of the world's 3.5 million patents.[11]

By 1973, postcolonial nations launched their agenda for a New International Economic Order at the Summit Conference of Non-Aligned Nations held in Algiers. Developing countries also called for a UN Code of Conduct on Transnational Corporations to better regulate the monopolistic power of transnational corporations.

Their demands were not met.

In 1974, WIPO concluded an agreement with the UN, establishing itself as the primary UN agency for all matters of intellectual property law. It is around this time that US industries painted competition from developing nations as "free-riding" on their R&D investments. It would become a battle cry, repeated ad nauseam to this day.

Like-minded leaders of major US corporations then mobilized to consolidate a US agenda for a trade-based conception of IP rights and to integrate IP into international trade policies. During this time, the Pharmaceutical Research Manufacturers Association, or PhRMA, a lobby group for pharmaceutical companies, emerged as a powerful and politically influential group.

The gospel of intellectual property was spread through business networks to chambers of commerce, trade associations, and every business council of import. Pfizer's CEO from 1972 to 1991, Edmund Pratt, had been raising concerns related to IP since the late 1970s, long before the HIV epidemic.[12] He referred to his involvement in framing the TRIPS Agreement as his greatest achievement. Ed Pratt was a broken record when it came to linking trade, investments, and intellectual property. He had been delivering speeches for nearly a decade in national and international platforms to lobby for stronger intellectual property rights, especially for pharmaceutical companies like Pfizer, which had huge markets in developing nations. Pfizer was among the first to raise concerns about "theft" and "piracy" of its IP property abroad.

On July 9, 1982, the *New York Times* carried an op-ed piece under the headline "Stealing from the Mind." The opinion piece was written by Barry MacTaggart, chairman of Pfizer International. The central argument was that American innovations were being stolen, and the culprits were countries like Brazil, India, and Mexico. For nearly three decades, starting in the 1970s, US corporations had been accusing Asian nations, India in particular, of piracy.

Pratt served on the Advisory Committee on Trade Negotiations for the Carter and Reagan administrations. In 1986, he cofounded the Intellectual Property Committee, which would go on to build relationships with industries across Europe and Japan, meet with WIPO officials, and lobby aggressively, all for the purpose of ensuring IP was included in trade negotiations.

He was not alone.

Representatives from many different sectors alleged that developing countries lacked vigilance in preventing the production of counterfeit goods and the unauthorized use of trademarks—while outsourcing environmentally polluting industries, such as pharmaceutical manufacturing, to nations like India and China.

Companies in the entertainment industry charged that developing countries were too tolerant of piracy of sound recordings and video, citing theoretical losses of billions of dollars per year. The persistent lobbying created fertile ground for a new set of laws aimed at arm-twisting the developing world. A core priority of large multinational companies was to ensure that the steps (to lower IP protection) taken in India, Brazil, Argentina, and Mexico would not set a precedent for other countries to follow.

Between 1981 and 1983, just as gay patients suffering from a rare form of pneumonia were turning up at hospitals in New York and Los Angeles, the North-South patent battle was heating up. Developing nations were intent on lowering the international minimum standards of patent protection, while developed countries were resolved to enhance them.

Once again, Goliath won.

The United States and the European Union bolstered their respective trade laws and gave themselves new unilateral tools to push for stronger IP protection in developing countries. Western nations used a combination of sticks, which came as unilateral threats, and carrots—promises of new market access for products of interest to developing countries.

Simultaneously, these tools were harnessed to pressure developing countries to accept the inclusion of IP rules in the General Agreement on Tariffs and Trade (GATT) regime.

From here, the tightening of the global IP regime was swift.

In 1981, the Caribbean Basic Economic Recovery Act elevated IP protection to one of the principal priorities of US trade policy. In 1984, the US Congress bolstered Section 301 of the US Trade and Tariff Act, authorizing the US government to rank trading partners based on the metrics of IP.

The countries that did not provide effective IP protection to American companies were placed on a "watch list" and threatened with trade sanctions. The watch list of transgressors, made by US trade representatives and compiled as the Special 301 report "remedied" what the US considered unfair trade practices by exerting constant pressure on developing nations to adhere to US standards or face sanctions.

With the revised Special 301 powers, the bully had fashioned himself a pulpit.

The US government began annual reviews of the IP practices of its trading partners, identifying countries that failed to provide adequate protection or fair and equitable market access for US nationals. The Special 301 provisions provoked an outcry from India and Brazil, who challenged the legality of US Special 301 actions for being aggressively extraterritorial. These standards were onerous for developing countries because they demanded far higher standards of IP protection than most would otherwise provide.

In 1982, Indian prime minister Indira Gandhi told the World Health Assembly, "The idea of a better ordered world is one in which medical discovery will be free of all patents and there will be no profiteering from life and death."

But world leaders were not listening.

Implicit in the new patent laws was that the US system was ideal, and the only correct solution was its IP laws. The Special 301 did not lay down norms or principles defining what "adequate" protection was. The implicit assumption was that anything different from that provided by US law was an unfair trade practice and inferior. By the mid-1980s, the US government started including IP provisions in its bilateral and regional agreements. US bilateral trade agreements with Israel (1985) and Vietnam (2000) were among the first to include IP commitments.

The European Union, as per Professor Peter Drahos, an Australian IP expert, was a "quiet free-rider" on the US.[13]

The combined force of the US and EU was a frontal attack on marginal gains, made through reforms, in the postcolonial world. Between 1985 and 1995, at least eighteen developing countries folded their cards and undertook reforms to strengthen patent protection on terms dictated by the US.

Industry lobbyists, like PhRMA, worked to enlist the support of European countries and Japan, building a fact-free case of the intrinsic ties between strong patent laws and development. The argument was that stronger laws helped poorer nations attract foreign investments, stimulated domestic innovation, and increased their global competitiveness. As industry and governments joined forces, the calls for TRIPS intensified.

In the US, the CEOs of twelve multinationals coordinated to sell the idea of TRIPS to Congress. In her political analysis of the emergence of the US position on TRIPS, Susan Sell documents how the pro-TRIPS agenda of US multinationals became not only the official policy of the US government but also the basis of the final TRIPS text.

In Geneva, the United States and the European Union insisted that IP be included in the Uruguay Round, the eighth round of multilateral trade negotiations (under GATT), spanning from 1986 to 1993, a vast trade negotiation between 123 countries.

The developing nations, a ragtag band, were walking into an ambush.

They arrived at the negotiation table disadvantaged, blindfolded, with arms firmly twisted behind their backs. The TRIPS Agreement was the kind of compromise that happens between the lion and the lamb. In contrast to the organized lobbying of the US and the EU, the developing nations were a small and loosely coordinated grouping of ten countries—Argentina, Brazil, Cuba, Egypt, India, Nicaragua, Nigeria, Peru, Tanzania, and Yugoslavia. The remaining developing countries either lacked resources or lacked technical knowledge of IP law at the birth of WTO and TRIPS. While developing nations were still wading through the technocratic and legal jargon, developed countries brought out many carrots and many more sticks.

The biggest stick was the Special 301 report.

By 1988, US Trade Representative announced the first findings of its Special 301 reviews. Ten developing countries were placed on the watch list, with threats of trade sanctions hanging over their heads, five of which were key countries opposing the US's IP agenda. Brazil and India, the greatest force of resistance during the Uruguay Round, were placed on the priority watch list.

India has remained there ever since.

In January 1989, the Group of 77 developing countries (G77) issued a collective statement saying the new IP laws were a "mere device and instrument for promoting the trade competitive interests of developed countries and their TransNational Corporations (TNCs)."[14]

The laws were protectionist, unfair, and only meant to safeguard the status quo of the world market, which guaranteed dominant positions to developed nations. The G77 issued a prescient warning, saying that this would, inevitably, lead to the "concentration of technological and economic power in the hands of the industrialized countries and in favour of their companies and TNCs and state-owned monopolies, thus perpetuating 'the technological gap between the technological haves and have-nots.'"[15]

The core group of resistors, thirteen countries (Argentina, Brazil, Chile, Colombia, Cuba, Egypt, India, Nigeria, Peru, Tanzania, and Uruguay, later joined by Pakistan and Zimbabwe), knew they had no choice but to accept TRIPS, however unfair. So they did the next best thing: submitted a detailed proposal designed to minimize the damage.

Cornered, the developing nations defended themselves the only way they could: by merging with what had been created with a few conditions squeezed in.

The West lost nothing.

It was decided that TRIPS would respect national legal systems, allow compulsory licenses in national emergency, and control anticompetitive practices. While the seven-year negotiations were underway, in 1991, the US initiated 301 proceedings against India, the staunchest critic of the TRIPS policy, followed by trade sanctions in 1992.

India held out longer than any other country in rejecting TRIPS but eventually caved in.

In her book, Carolyn Deere noted that industries that had lobbied for TRIPS were among the world's largest and most profitable: the US$650 billion per year global pharmaceutical industry (estimated to increase to $US900 billion in the next four years), the commercial seed industry (worth an estimated US$21 billion per year), and the global software and entertainment industries (worth an estimated US$800 billion per year). US companies in these sectors would go on to dominate global markets, with the TRIPS patent protection at the heart of their business model.

According to a 2002 World Bank estimate, Brazil lost US$530 million, China US$5.1 billion, India US$903 million, and the Republic of Korea US$15.3 billion because of TRIPS.

The law brought dizzying profits to pharmaceutical companies and, in that process, contributed to a rise in drug prices within the US. In the developing world, it put new, lifesaving drugs in a stranglehold, creating "clinical deserts" most visibly during the HIV/AIDS crisis, which was peaking as the TRIPS Agreement was being drafted.

Not coincidentally, Bill Gates would emerge as the world's richest man just as WTO TRIPS went into effect, chaining the developing world in knowledge monopolies. He would establish the Bill and Melinda Gates Foundation in the summer of 1999.

In 2005, the United States alone earned US$33 billion due to IP enforcement, more than its total development assistance budget of US$27 billion for that year. The rich were giving from one hand, taking back with interest with the other. The new laws would speed the transfer of capital from developing to developed countries and exacerbate global inequities, especially in health, leading to unconscionable loss of life in developing nations.

Amid growing debates on globalization, TRIPS—the most important law on knowledge monopoly in the twenty-first century—was a symbol both of the vulnerability of postcolonial nations and of the coercive pressures from developed countries. It was included as one of the WTO's core agreements despite consistent opposition from developing countries.

Fewer than 20 of the 106 developing countries who were members of the WTO were involved in the negotiations. Once again, the colonies were not at the negotiating table.

On January 1, 1995, the WHO, with its shiny new TRIPS law, replaced the GATT regime.

The fight for access to AIDS medicines hit a crescendo in 1995 when WTO was created, and the TRIPS Agreement created the obligation for all WTO members to grant patents with a minimum of twenty years.[16] This was also the moment when HIV activists from ACT UP and other organizations were occupying Wall Street and opposing high drug prices.

For the first time, IP was framed in "patents versus patients" terms.

The demand to do something about the outrageous law grew louder and louder right after developed nations imposed it. The TRIPS Agreement was negotiated without any involvement of the health community. It was a one-size-fits-all policy that did not distinguish between lifesaving medicines, movies, refrigerators, and iPhones.

The policy would haunt American patients just as much as it haunted poor nations.

With drugs protected under patent monopolies, pharmaceutical companies started pricing at will. In a perfect example of capitalism devouring its own, American pharmaceutical companies, after conquering the rest of the world, turned on their own citizens. While they outsourced drug manufacturing to India (Johnson & Johnson manufactured bedaquiline in India, at a fraction of the US cost), they continued to charge exorbitant prices in domestic markets. Armed with TRIPS, Big Pharma was able to flex its muscles all over the world.

One case, in particular, stood out.

In 1998, reeling under HIV, the South African government was exploring changes to its Patents Act so that it could import affordable generic drugs. In December 1997, Nelson Mandela's government passed a law giving the health ministry powers to produce, purchase, and import low-cost drugs, including unbranded versions of combination therapies priced by Western drug companies at \$10,000 and more.

The changes were opposed by the multinational drug companies during their passage through parliament. In a ruthless and infamous move, forty pharmaceutical companies took the South African government to court to try to stop it from enacting legislation aimed at reducing the price of medicines. It was a test case with international implications.

The pharmaceutical companies accused the South African government of "parallel importing"—importing without the permission of the intellectual property owner of the drug. The resulting controversy, and the South African government's battle with Big Pharma over HIV medicines, led to the "Doha Declaration," a genuine milestone in public health that recognized "the gravity of the public health problems afflicting many developing and least developed countries, especially those resulting from HIV/AIDS, tuberculosis, malaria and other epidemics" and affirmed "that the [TRIPS] Agreement does not and should not prevent Members from taking measures to protect public health."[17]

The case, brought by forty pharma companies, was withdrawn in 2001, a few months after Cipla offered the drugs at a dollar a day, leading to a public relations nightmare for pharmaceutical companies, which could no longer say they could not afford to help.[18] The companies dropped their lawsuit and waived their patents, and generic HIV drugs began to flow into Africa.

The Doha Declaration was just as important as the Durban Declaration a year earlier. It gave countries practical tools and political confidence to overcome patent barriers and access medicines.

It offered a new way of thinking about patents and medicines.

CHAPTER 11

────◆────

THE BUSINESS OF DYING

A large part of being sick is having to watch your family watch you be sick. That's where Nandita Venkatesan was in 2013. She has a face that even strangers see and smile at. Her short crop of hair, as far as I can tell, is always ruffled.

Over the course of five years, she would face one personal blow after another. She would be diagnosed with tuberculosis. Be cured. Relapse. Lose her hearing. Lose friends. Lose her family home.

Nandita spent a decade battling a wretched bacterium and an even more wretched health system. In the end, she gained more than she lost. The experience was a crucible from which she emerged an able leader, forged in crisis.

She had grown up in Thane, a middle-class neighborhood in suburban Mumbai, with her younger brother, Niranjan, whom she calls Ninja. Their home had a lot of rules. There were set times to get up, to study, to offer prayers, and to play, and their life moved in these predictable rhythms. The parents—her father, a chartered accountant, and her mother, an economics lecturer—had clear

expectations for the children when it came to academic performance. Shoddiness in school was unacceptable.

Amid all this, bharata natyam, a classical Hindu dance form,
was her steady love. The dance form comes from the temples of
southern India, and the name translates to "India's dance." She
had grown up loving classical dance and spent years training
in it.

An enlarged still from a solo performance occupies a place of
pride in the family's apartment in Thane. She is in full costume,
with anklets, kohl-rimmed eyes, and fine flowing silk with pleats
designed to glide with her body. Her face is glowing, and she is
maintaining an elegant posture that could very well belong to one
of those panels carved into the temples of southern India.

As a child, she never wanted for the basics: health, education, and safety. Her future was charted. After her graduation, she
would enroll in whatever higher education she wanted to pursue,
and then her parents would find her a suitable boy—unless she
came home with an acceptable choice.

Overall, life was predictable and steadily happy, and she never
felt unsafe, growing up under the careful gaze of her parents.

That lasted until May 2007, when she had her first brush with
TB, starting her decade-long struggle with the bacteria. She would
relapse on November 22, 2013, two days after her twenty-fourth
birthday.

She remembers everything about that day—a slow-motion
train wreck that would remain burned into her brain. The date
is now marked on her calendar, and she sees it approaching each
year, measuring life in the distance she has managed to put between
herself and that day.

That afternoon she decided to take a short nap. When she woke up after ten minutes, she could not hear anything.

She looked around and saw that her mother, Veena, was talking to Ninja. She could see their mouths move but could not hear a thing. She went to her phone, plugged her earphones in, and played some music.

"I could *see* the song was playing, but I could not hear it," she says.

The deafness was the side effect of a toxic antibiotic injection, kanamycin (pronounced "can-a-my-sin"). The drug would not get marketing approval by today's safety standards. It is an old drug that mutilates the body; one in four patients go deaf.

Nandita happened to be the fourth patient.

In 2013, four years after she was cured of drug-sensitive TB, it became clear that she had drug-resistant TB. A team of private doctors were treating her. The surgeon was a gastroenterologist, the physician was an expert in TB, and the one prescribing medicine was a regular physician. They had put her on kanamycin, used to treat serious bacterial infections in different parts of the body. But it is for short-term use only (usually seven to ten days), and she had been on the injectable for months.

Kanamycin's extensive side effects include neuromuscular blockade, hair cell damage, and ototoxicity (audiotoxicity), which can cause irreversible or partially reversible bilateral hearing loss.

"Two days after my birthday, I had lost my hearing," she told me in April 2019, over chai and sandwiches.

"On both sides, the level of deafness was profound. The left side was 100 percent, and the right side was between 50 and 60 percent. But it was gradually going down, and then it reached 90 percent. By 2016, within two years' time, I was profoundly deaf in both ears."

Profoundly deaf.

Those words hung over her like a thick miasma.

In the previous months, between June and September 2013, she had undergone four lifesaving surgeries. All were dramatic admissions—the kind where the patient falls to the floor, unresponsive, and no one knows if they will survive. Each time, she was rushed to the hospital, propped on to a gurney, and attached to numerous tubes and machines that made her mother's heart sink faster than a stone.

All four were emergency surgeries, back-to-back.

"I had a relapse. I was trying some medicines, and each time the doctors would turn to surgery because the medicines were not working."

Her weight was going down fast. She was all knees and elbows, gaunt beyond recognition, a mere shadow of the glowing face dancing in the photo in her living room.

The relapse was from intestinal drug-resistant tuberculosis. Yes, you can get TB in your intestines. When the infection is not in the lungs, it is called extrapulmonary tuberculosis.

It is not infectious, but it is dangerous.

"I was constantly breathless and collapsed at home. I was not regaining consciousness, so I was back in the hospital, being fed intravenously for the next two months. I did not eat food for two months," she adds.

The business of dying is extremely specific.

In her case, it meant that she was in bed, hooked to tubes carrying a milky white substance that gave her body the nutrients it needed. She was allowed only twenty-five-milliliter sips of water, once every five hours. She was thin to begin with, and the relapse meant that in a couple of months, she lost twenty-three kilograms (roughly fifty pounds). Her hair started to thin, as is usually the case with extreme undernourishment. "I vividly remember going for a small walk in the hospital and seeing a reflection of myself in a glass window—with bald patches. I couldn't recognise myself," she told the *Hindu* in an interview in 2016.[1] There is a photo of her from this time, all ribs, knees, and elbows.

That's what having a *curable* disease looks like, she thought.

Her first brush with TB, the drug-sensitive kind, was in November 2007, a month after she began her undergraduate course at Ruia College in Matunga, in central Mumbai. She had seen three different doctors and spent ninety days in search of the correct diagnosis. After diagnosis, the first piece of advice from her treating physician—a private doctor—was not to tell her friends about her condition. "She told me my friends 'might stay away' if I was honest about my TB diagnosis."

Even from the doctor's perspective, she says, TB was something to be ashamed of. "The doctor *taught* me to be ashamed. I did not even have a kind of TB that was contagious," she said.

TB treatment, much like cancer treatment, is rough.

Over the next fifteen months, Nandita would go on the same thousand-pill odyssey every TB patient endures. TB treatment places a huge "pill burden" on patients. Ingesting ten to fifteen powerful drugs at the exact same time, day after day, for months is not easy. Then the side effects show up, starting with dead taste buds.

It was difficult, but she learned to live with it—the fistfuls of pills, the gnawing pain in her stomach, extreme exhaustion, and intense fury at having caught the infection. Through this period, she kept her head down, did everything by the book, and was cured.

For the next few years, life went on. She graduated, moved to Delhi to do her postgraduate work in journalism, and made friends.

She was in her element.

That was when her TB relapsed, in May 2013.

She had lulled herself into thinking TB was in her past when the familiar gnawing pain in the stomach returned. It completely blindsided her. For days she was in shock, followed by weeks of denial. By November, she had lost her hearing.

The next few years hit like wave upon wave of torrential grief for her and for her family, who had a helpless ringside seat in this nightmare.

Her mother quit her job to take care of her progressively worsening child. The relapse affected Ninja too. Some family photos from that time reveal the chaos that had engulfed the household—swollen eyes, haunted faces, and an exhaustion as profound as Nandita's deafness. In some photos, Nandita looks like someone who hasn't slept in weeks, a common side effect of the toxic medicines.

"There was no part of the day when I was not crying," she told me, sipping her chai and working on her sandwich.

Then came the monster side effect, unfortunately common in TB patients: depression. A patient suffering from TB-related depression once described it as being "pinned to the floor of an ocean" while watching the world enjoying a day at the beach. That's how life felt for Nandita. The world seemed to not care as her life disintegrated.

"There was a time between December and April of the year [2014] . . ." She begins the sentence, but her voice trails away. A few seconds later, she picks it up elsewhere. "I used to cry fourteen hours at a stretch, nonstop."

She cried so much it altered her sleep cycle. She cried all night, slept from 6:00 a.m. to noon, woke up, cried more, passed out, and repeated the cycle—a caricature of a terminal patient.

"I was in horrifying pain. Thinking about it gives me goose-bumps even now. I'd keep on crying, and the physical pain, without my knowledge, transformed into a severe form of depression." Her depression manifested in many ways, one of which was suicidal ideation.

"I felt invisible. The world that just kept going without even noticing this had happened to me," she said. It is inexplicable that TB patients, unlike cancer patients, are expected to overcome a diagnosis without support groups, counseling, or empathy from doctors.

Instead, they get a steady stream of stigma and shame.

Weeks turned into months, and months turned into years. She had not left her bed. The few times she tried to step out for a trip to the hospital, her eyes could no longer adjust to the sun.

Meanwhile, the deafness was causing unbearable heartache to her family. They had made quite a few adjustments; there was now a bulb that lit up when the doorbell rang. No one would receive phone calls if she was in the same room, knowing they could agitate her. She'd put her earplugs in, sit in a corner of her room, and pretend that she could hear. Dancing was out of the question.

"I kept thinking, How come things went so wrong for me? I'd scream at my family for pulling out their phones in front of me. I'd tried to end my life." Thankfully, Ninja was home when she tried; he saw her and stopped her just in time.

For the next two years, between 2013 and 2015, the family hurtled from one crisis to another. Treatment expenses were mounting, and they had to sell their house. "We could not manage the finances anymore. We sold our house. That was a big blow for me. I did not expect it at all. It was *our* house—the biggest investment of my parents' lives. They are in their fifties. You don't expect, at that point in your life, to not have a roof over your head," she said.

Her family moved to an apartment in the same suburban neighborhood where they'd lived all their lives. The smaller two-bedroom apartment in Thane had everything they needed. "With the money, we paid off medical debt and kept some money aside for Ninja's education. We put the rest into my treatment," she told me. Her health insurance covered treatment worth US$13,000. The expenses were much more than that. The treatment costs were around US$60,000.

She pulls out a diary entry from the day her family vacated their home. On moving day, she noticed her brother, father, and mother were mostly silent. "The silence was not from my deafness. It was from the heaviness of having to sell the house," the diary entry reads.

Through this period, she was a meticulous soldier when it came to adhering to doctor's orders. She took her pills, ate well, and hoped to catch a break.

"It was the lowest point in this entire saga for me," she said.

The good news, however, was that she had reached the bottom of the seemingly bottomless pit.

She was not dying.

And since she was alive, she thought she might as well dance. She could not hear a thing and barely had the stamina to stay upright, but she decided to put on her anklets, converted the beats into numbers, and got on stage in October 2015.

"It was a five-minute performance; I did not have more strength than that. But it got me to a place where I felt hope again for the first time in years," she said.

She had not danced in three years.

By April 2016, she had found a job with *Economic Times*, one of India's biggest financial newspapers and among the few organizations to employee people with disabilities. At work, she confronted her worst fears. "I'd see people talking on the phone, run to the bathroom, and cry in the stalls. I'd break down all the time. I felt so helpless every time someone received a phone call. It was mocking me."

She was still dealing with side effects as well. In 2016, when she finally started getting out in the sun, she got severe headaches and nausea. Lying in bed for years at a stretch meant she had twisted her left leg. "The muscles in one of my legs had changed from not being used. I had to practice walking again. All of this is also TB, but no one talks about that aspect of the disease."

Eventually, she learned to be patient with herself.

In April 2016, she was struggling to adjust in her new job, still going back and forth with her doctors to manage her medications' side effects. But things were starting to look up. That's when she noticed the reporting about TB in Indian newspapers. She was stuck in a "frequency illusion"—when you know something others don't, and you start seeing it everywhere.

As a trained journalist, she was unable to grasp why TB was reported on so poorly. "The press coverage reduced the epidemic to a number, without telling any real stories about the people suffering. What has happened to me is *so dangerous*; why is it not being covered that way?" She could not stand being reduced to a statistic. "Two million cases? Those are two million people. I was one of those people. I was bothered that there were no stories behind those numbers. I had to do something," she told me.

She pulled out a diary from her cupboard and opened it to a page where she had posed her questions to her doctor. The doctor had responded, "Why don't *you* talk about it? Make a support group for patients, or start a blog."

That was the first time she thought about TB advocacy.

In January 2016, a website called YourStory carried her experience under this headline: "Tuberculosis Took Away 22kg and Most of Her Hearing, but Nandita Continues to Dance to the Music of Life."[2] It went viral in TB circles.

With three thousand shares, it reached a large number of TB patients or relatives. Fellow TB patients started reaching out to her on Facebook. The advocacy began with her helping a couple of people, telling them they would be fine. Soon, more and more patients contacted her.

This was the first time she had openly admitted to having lived with TB. So far, except with her immediate family and a few friends, she had been vague about the nature of her illness. Her first doctor's stigmatizing advice to hide her diagnosis was difficult to shake off.

Later in 2016, she googled her YourStory article out of curiosity. Dr. Pai—who was vocal and active on social media platforms—had shared it.

That's how she met him—via Twitter.

"I started considering advocacy. I went to a couple of places to speak about my experience and became a voice in TB circles. I started telling patients and policy makers alike that they could reach out to me if they need a patient's perspective," she recalls.

By June 2017, she had given a TEDx Talk on hearing loss from toxic TB drugs and life after TB.[3] Dr. Pai invited her to McGill University in Montreal to share her experiences at the McGill Summer Institute in Infectious Diseases and Global Health. In fact, Dr. Pai decided to open the course by asking the survivors to speak on why good diagnosis matters to patients.

"A test result to check drug resistance takes six weeks to come. But that time is enough to turn a patient's life upside down!" Nandita told the room full of aspiring doctors.

The decision to invite survivors absolutely shook up everyone in the first thirty minutes of class, Dr. Pai said. "Sometimes we call survivors toward the end of the course. This wasn't like that. I gave them the first hour of the course. Nandita had them [the students] in tears. It totally changed the rest of the course. The impact they had was beyond dramatic. Next year we invited more survivors. We are steadily stepping it up each year," said Dr. Pai.

I asked Dr. Pai why he invited TB survivors to Montreal.

He said he was making up for lost time. "I am the first one to admit I woke up late in my life. For the first ten years of my life as a TB researcher, I worked without involving patients. Obviously, I knew about the importance of civil society. I just did not internalize it. They need to be at the center of the discussion. I had been looking at HIV. Slowly, I realized they [the HIV movement] did amazing things in the past because they were fueled by energy and activism of the patients," he says.

For a long time, India's National TB Elimination Program (NTEP), was unaware that deafness was a side effect of the antibiotics being prescribed to TB patients in India. "When I started speaking up about this at government meetings, officials were always surprised. They looked puzzled. The fact that such a high degree of hearing loss is happening and the people who run the TB policy do not even know but continue to roll out toxic drugs is so scary," she told me.

Nandita was shocked.

"I lost my hearing because of them—*and they don't even know!* No one is collecting this data. I tried searching for data on audiotoxicity of kanamycin injections." She found nothing. The Indian government has been doling out an old, toxic medicine without collecting any data on how it maimed patients.

"A huge number of people have lost hearing from a drug distributed by the government, under a national policy. Unless data is collected, how will they understand the level of crisis? I feel angry about this," she added.

When I asked Nandita why she is not simply moving on and forgetting all about TB, she said, "I wouldn't wish anyone to go through what I did with DR TB. We cannot let more patients go deaf."

She fought TB twice and eventually lived to tell the tale. In 2018, she got her first all-clear test results. As the disease faded into the past, she thrived. She went back to dancing while working full time. There were other victories too. She addressed the 2018 United Nations General Assembly, the first-ever such meeting on tuberculosis, where she told the heads of state to stop treating patients with outdated and toxic antibiotics. The TB community passed the hat around, and she was able to get cochlear implants in February 2019. It was a big day within the TB community, and she exchanged celebratory messages with many.

She shared a recording of her hearing for the first time after the implants. When it was switched on, she said, "I first heard my audiologist. He wrote to me that he had switched on the device and that I was going to hear something.

"Then he asked, 'How am I sounding?'"

She stared in amazement as the thrill of it began to make its way through her. For the TB community, it was one of those rare days when something hopeful had happened. The first person she spoke to was her mother.

There was more good news.

She received the Chevening/Weidenfeld-Hoffman Trust Scholarship in 2020 to study public policy at Keble College, Oxford University, with a special focus on health.

I asked her what she dreams of now. Is this her happy ending?

She smiled radiantly and surprised me with a well-thought-out dream sequence: "Everybody who died of TB comes back to celebrate when all patients have access to new treatments. I'd be an ex-TB activist; I'd do something else . . . not sure what."

CHAPTER 12

THE PHANTOM PLAGUE AND THE MISSING MILLIONS

The WHO estimates that one-*fourth* of the world's population has latent TB.

The HIV epidemic was a rude awakening.

Suddenly there was a realization that TB was a grave crisis. HIV, because it compromised immunity, liberated the latent TB. The logic was inescapable: any widespread epidemic that adversely affected immunity had the capacity to make latent TB into an active and deadly killer.

In Mumbai, TB is everywhere and nowhere.

Spotting the bacteria is not unlike spotting a tiger in a jungle— while glimpses are uncommon or fleeting, there are fresh prints that show a predator is lurking nearby. You don't have to walk into hospitals to find it. You see it in spit stains all over the city, in the unprotected coughing and sneezing in crowded buses, in tightly packed ghettos. Today, India is a moist "nation of spitters."

The spread of TB is extensive. And it is extensively denied.

Indian TB patients are in the same situation South African patients diagnosed with HIV/AIDS in the 1990s were: the epidemic is at its peak, and the drugs are not available. The Indian government is engaging in TB denialism with as much fervor as the South African government once did. TB has become a twenty-first-century disease being fought with (for the most part) nineteenth-century tools.

In India, these medieval tools are wielded by an army of science-deficient doctors for a government with scant respect for science, each piling errors on errors.

According to the WHO, the first case of *extensively* drug-resistant tuberculosis was reported in 2006 in Italy. In 2009, fifteen TB patients in Iran were diagnosed with the same strain. In December 2011, Mumbai doctors reported four patients, and a few weeks later, the *Times of India* reported eight more cases in Mumbai. The WHO took a while, as is customary, before settling on calling it XDR TB. Meanwhile, scientists in different parts of the world were using new terms like "XXDR TB," "super XDR TB," and "totally drug-resistant TB" ("TDR TB") interchangeably.

In Mumbai, Dr. Udwadia was calling it TDR TB.

He had treated the four patients in 2011 and, methodical as he is, wrote a paper about the new, untreatable *avatar* of TB.[1] He and his colleagues called the strain TDR TB, the term coined in 2009 by Iranian doctors who had treated the fifteen patients showing no response to the first- and second-line antibiotics. Dr. Udwadia's paper warned of an antibiotic apocalypse, when there will be no drugs known to modern medicine that could cure these emerging strains of the bacteria.

The Indian government did not like the prognosis.

It raided his lab, seized the patient samples, and pressured Dr. Udwadia to retract the paper.[2] The NTEP did everything it could to sweep this piece of bad news under the rug. The tidal wave of bureaucracy rolled over the unimpeachable scientific evidence and once again drowned the science out in the twenty-first century as it had in the nineteenth. The Indian government's response to new data on TDR TB had the same hallmarks of ignorance and arrogance that Ignaz Semmelweis dealt with.

Dr. Udwadia has spent years speaking up to an increasingly unreasonable government.

He has a skeptical squint and a wry smile that redoubles the sense of skepticism. "They came down on us like a ton of bricks. Their first response was denial. Their second response was to take away our samples," remembered Dr. Udwadia, still surprised at the government's reaction, years later.

He and his employers at the Hinduja Hospital were accused of spreading panic by using the term "totally drug resistant." The Indian government argued that no such term had been approved by the WHO.[3] Then, the NTEP dismissed his findings because the Hinduja Hospital's laboratory—one of the finest in the country—had not been accredited by the government. So, their word could not be taken seriously. The government refused to investigate any further. But global media was starting to cover the story, so the ministry needed to be seen to run their own tests. "Literally, they seized culture from our laboratories. They took them for cross-checking," says Dr. Udwadia.

His epic struggle against TB and the Indian government's vast labyrinth of bureaucracy was reported in the *New York Times* in September 2016.[4]

* * *

The study in which actors were trained to walk into a doctor's clinic with every red-flag symptom of TB has since been replicated in three other countries: South Africa, China, and Kenya. The "patients" all report a persistent fever and cough for two weeks, the first red flag. Then they follow a set script:

> **Regular Jane Doctor:** Do you have cough with phlegm?
> **RJ Actor-Patient:** Yes.
> Fever?
> Yes.
> Weight loss?
> Yes.
> Loss of appetite?
> Yes.

This is the textbook definition of a patient who should be screened for a TB test. In all the participating countries, the study discovered three alarming failures:

1. Most doctors could not correctly diagnose TB patients.
2. Even if they did, they did not correctly treat them.
3. Without proper medical guidance, the patients—all falling through the cracks of the health-care system—continued to infect their loved ones.

The number of undetected TB cases is genuinely alarming. Within global health, this problem has come to be known as "the missing millions." According to the WHO, in 2019, 10 million people fell ill with TB. Only 7.1 million were picked up by national TB treatment programs. So 2.9 million were either undetected or unreported.

You cannot treat what you cannot diagnose.

The study found that across all four countries—India, South Africa, China, and Kenya—only 35 percent of the actor-patients were "correctly managed."[5] To begin with, researchers had set a low bar for the definition of "correctly managed." "If the doctor referred the patient to another doctor or referred her to a government hospital—instead of screening her—we accepted it as a 'correct diagnosis.' We accepted any screening test they recommended as well—x-rays, sputum smears, and Gene Xpert. It was broadly defined," Dr. Pai told me in a Skype interview.

Even using this lenient definition, only one in five actor-patients was correctly managed. In Mumbai, 37 percent of patients were correctly managed, Nairobi 33 percent, rural China 28–38 percent, and South Africa, the "best" performer, 43 percent.

At this stage the study team was not looking at *what was being prescribed* but simply trying to see if doctors could diagnose TB correctly. The treatment, when it was recognized as necessary, often compounded the problem: "What they [doctors who've correctly diagnosed their patients] end up doing is, hit them with multiple rounds of broad-spectrum antibiotics."

Basically, the few patients who are diagnosed correctly are carpet-bombed with powerful antibiotics, cough syrups, steroids, and antihistamines to see what "works." Doctors, especially those in the private sector, were throwing a bunch of pills at the bacteria, found Dr. Pai. "An average prescription has four to five pills, and the doctors say come back in two weeks if it doesn't get better," Dr Pai told me in 2019.

Only 10 percent of the actor-patients were referred to specialists, as they should have been immediately. "The job of the primary care doctor seems to be to retain the patient. At this stage, referral is practically dead," the study concluded.[6]

In the private sector—where retaining the patient is more important than treating them—doctors send back patients, asking them to try antibiotics for a couple of weeks, leaving them to infect others during this period.

The hellish cycle of misdiagnosis can last for weeks as the patient is bounced from one doctor to another, feeling increasingly worse: "In most parts of the world, TB is only diagnosed after about three rounds of this. . . . Patients start with pharmacy, go to traditional medicine, switch to allopathy, change doctors," Dr. Pai told me.

Thanks to the study, we now know it takes a TB patient an average of sixty days and a minimum of three doctors to receive correct treatment. During this diagnostic delay, patients are actively infectious.

Government hospitals at least keep records.

India is, not coincidentally, home to one of the largest unregulated private sectors in the world, a vast and unregulated mess whose raison d'être has been to undercut the government-run, taxpayer-funded health system.

In April 2019, Dr. Pai described the discrepant numbers regarding undetected or unreported TB to an audience at the London School of Hygiene and Tropical Medicines: "The missing could either be because they are walking around, undiagnosed. Or they are seeking care at pharmacies, or at private clinics. My hunch says that the missing patients are diagnosed but not reported. The countries with the most privatized health care are not only the ones with the largest patient burden but also the ones with the most missing patients. There is a clear correlation between private care seeking and the missing millions. That's why working with the private sector is so critical, especially for India," explained Dr. Pai.

Global TB experts, including Dr. Pai, reviewed thirty-two national tuberculosis surveys done in twenty-six countries between 2000 and 2016. All surveys revealed that, globally, everyone had underestimated the prevalence of TB.

It was a phantom plague.

In October 2016, the WHO said it had seriously underestimated the global TB epidemic because of inaccurate estimates of the tuberculosis burden in India between 2000 and 2015.[7] The most alarming finding of the latest Global TB Report 2016 was that India had reported only 56 percent of its TB burden in 2014 and 59 percent in 2015. The massive underestimating resulted in the WHO revising the global TB burden upward by over four million cases.[8]

The same problem occurred in all seven countries with the most TB patients in the world—India, Indonesia, China, the Philippines, Pakistan, Nigeria, and South Africa.

Speaking to me on the condition of anonymity, a senior bureaucrat in the health ministry was clear about the prospects of meeting Modi's ambitious 2025 target to eliminate TB: "We did not give this target. This was set by nontechnical people. If you are asking me whether we will end TB by 2025, the answer is simple: we will not."

To "end TB" by 2025, India would have to bring down new infections from the current 204 per one million people to 40. "This cannot even be done by 2040, if all hands were on deck, and the policy had no budget constraints," the official added.

* * *

India is not alone in failing to meet its ambitions to eliminate TB.

In 1993 to 1994, whiplashed by the surge in TB cases that was brought on by the HIV epidemic, WHO announced the DOTS program to control TB.[9] The World Bank made support of TB programs contingent on the adoption of DOTS, and the gospel of DOTS spread far and wide. Twenty years after its introduction, it had become clear that the DOTS strategy was one of the WHO's more spectacular failures.

Until 2006, DOTS was the recommended approach to global TB control.[10] When they found DR TB, DOTS recommended *retreatment*, with the *same* cocktail of drugs that had not worked in the first place, adding to the disease's resistance. The doses were insufficient to treat and cure TB but enough to boost antibiotic resistance in the bacteria. "The various iterations of DOTS were all about 'KISS'—keep it simple, stupid," said Dr. Paul Farmer, medical anthropologist and chair of the Department of Global Health and Social Medicine at Harvard Medical School since 2009. In 1987, Dr. Farmer helped found a nonprofit called Partners in Health to provide quality medical care, including treatment for tuberculosis, in rural central Haiti. The international organization now works in eleven countries and serves millions of patients with a clear medical and moral vision: to privilege effectiveness rather than cost-effectiveness.

Dr. Farmer's organization takes a moral stand against the "control-over-care" paradigm, where disease control is more important than caring for patients. "TB is where this paradigm has had especially devastating effects. The 'care question' is an entirely different conversation from the 'control question,'" Dr. Farmer told me over Zoom in February 2021. He added that TB policy is often misguided, in part because it often deems treatment (especially of drug-resistant strains) too costly, complex, and unsustainable for the poor.

Writing for the *Lancet* in September 2021, Professor Furin said the same thing but in a different way. "In such parlance, human beings are reduced to disability-adjusted life-years and suffering is only worth addressing if doing so is deemed to be sustainable or cost-effective," she wrote about the language of public health.[11]

To put it in nonmedical terms, TB policies are a failure because of the moral foundation prioritizing cost of care over care itself—a flaw from which other flaws originate, especially those in budgeting. "In 2017, an estimated US$10.9 billion was spent on tuberculosis compared with $20.2 billion spent on HIV. The Stop TB Partnership has estimated a $7 billion shortfall in tuberculosis funding per year," the *Lancet* piece noted.[12]

At some point toward the end of the 1990s, health experts realized that the DOTS program could fuel a DR TB epidemic.

In 1999, experts in Geneva went back to the drawing board and came up with a new DOTS-Plus strategy. In 2001, as the first DOTS-Plus pilot projects were launched, the WHO set up the Stop TB Partnership in Geneva, a dedicated vertical to control the spiraling global epidemic. They also set up the Global Drug Facility in Geneva, with the express purpose of purchasing antibiotics for poor nations where TB was ripping through communities.

One of the biggest challenges facing DOTS-Plus was that there were no new antibiotics left. Twenty years ago, Dr. Farmer was presenting a paper on patients who were developing resistance to first-line TB drugs. "At the end of it, someone came up to me and said, 'If you are right, that means we have to reframe all of our guidelines.' And then added, 'But we just printed the guidelines!'"

Dr. Farmer defines this approach as one of a "public health luddite"—the kind of person who resists tests because that would reveal more drug resistance. "They are supposed to be on our team. But they keep us from imagining a world in which DOTS is about the shortest, most effective, symptom-free therapy we can recommend for our patients. Instead, we face numerous situations where countries do not even want to discover new clusters of drug-resistant disease."

By 2000, global TB targets set in 1991 had still not been met. So, more international meetings were held, and a new Amsterdam Declaration to Stop TB aimed at the same goals, but this time to be achieved by 2005.

"At these TB meetings, we [the public health community] reliably talk about the same thing over and over again. There is no discussion of new vaccines, new diagnostics, new therapies. These low aspirations are driving doctors like Zarir [Dr. Udwadia] and me crazy. Not the pathogens or the lack of medicines—that's bad enough—but our chief antagonists tend to be public health luddites. My frustration is with their unambitious approach," Dr. Farmer told me in February 2021 over Zoom.

When 2006 rolled in, the 1991 targets set in the Global Plan to Stop TB had still not been reached.

Predictably, more international meetings were held, and another global plan was hatched, this time for 2006–2015. This time targets were woven into the Millennium Development Goals. The Global Plan was subsequently updated in 2010, to become the Global Plan to Stop TB 2011–2015. Dependably, 2015 came and went without any global targets being met.

This time, after more conferences, a plan was hatched to "End TB" by 2030.

Meetings were held, documents were written, and targets were set. Terms like "paradigm shift" and "radical change" were thrown around, and there was a notion that this time it was different.

Every shred of evidence from the most affected parts of the world showed that it was more of the same. As the disease spread, policy experts were behaving like luddites once again. "A blind commitment to a DOTS regimen was the policy decision of a luddite, of those who felt we must preserve antibiotics for the sake of preserving them rather than of making use of them in service of our patients. This is a socialization of scarcity, and it comes from— not clinicians or pharmaceutical companies or patients—but from many development economists and public health experts.

"We know all drug resistance is generally a result of human actions. But are patients really at fault? I don't think so, and I know Dr. Udwadia doesn't. Many TB 'experts' blamed patients for lack of adherence, when they really should have been interrogating the programs professing to serve them," Dr. Farmer told me.

In March 2019, the *Lancet* dedicated an issue to tuberculosis. The first sentence read, "Tuberculosis can be treated, prevented, and cured." Commenting on the failure of the DOTS policy, the *Lancet* noted the biggest shortcomings of the policy were "reliance on a simplified one-size-fits-all approach that did not meet the different needs of individual patients, HIV co-infection and the spread of drug-resistant TB, and the huge reservoir of latent TB infections."

It was a tragic understatement, especially about the scale of latent TB infection.

When people with a strong immune system are infected, the TB bacteria typically gets "walled off." When a body is unable to eliminate the bacteria, it isolates it by forming a granuloma, a collection of immune cells that make sure it doesn't replicate. The TB bacteria can stay imprisoned like this for up to forty years. As a patient's immunity fails or as they age, the wall crumbles and the bacteria break out.

So how much latent TB is there in the world?

We don't know—much the same way as we don't know how many millions of patients are missing because no one is looking for them.

What we do know for sure is that latent TB patients are a warehouse of future TB patients.

* * *

TB activism, globally and in India, has not managed to unify in ways that are threatening to its adversaries: pharmaceutical companies and public health luddites. TB activism in India, as well as around the world, has been fragmented.

That is changing.

Patient survivors in high-burden countries are now demanding a seat at the negotiating table. In India, after successfully completing treatment for XDR TB, twenty-four-year-old Nandita emerged as a leading voice. "Esteemed heads of state, you must act now. Your declaration will make a difference only if it is backed by action. . . . I cannot hear you today. But I will make sure you hear me, loud and clear."[13]

She was speaking at the UN General Assembly meeting on TB and demanding a shorter treatment regimen, removal of toxic injectables (like the kanamycin that made her deaf), and access to new medicines like bedaquiline and delamanid. While doling out medicines that are making patients deaf, the government has been rationing a much safer drug—bedaquiline—on grounds that it *might have* cardiotoxicity.

It does not.

The latest studies show that not a single patient on bedaquiline has been lost due to cardiotoxicity of the drug, anywhere in the world.

"How can you care about cardiotoxicity in bedaquiline but not about audiotoxicity in kanamycin? We now have data that cardiotoxicity fears were overstated. Why are we not using the best medicines? Phumeza and I are living examples of how horrible the current drugs are," Nandita would ask me later, when we met in Mumbai in April 2019. She was referring to her friend and fellow survivor, Phumeza Tisile from Khayelitsha, Cape Town, South Africa. The two went through tragedies that were continents apart but had nearly identical details; they are two of the many survivors who have coalesced into a strong, close-knit community that is taking on Big Pharma. In these communities, survivor-patients exchange their stories, riff off each other, and form strong bonds based entirely on the shared trauma of having gone through TB treatment.

Exactly like Dr. Pai's actor-patient study predicted, Tisile was poorly diagnosed at age nineteen and mistreated. Doctors put her on kanamycin, which made her deaf.

Like Nandita, the drug robbed her of hearing without doing anything to help cure TB. Tisile was put on a twenty-thousand-pill odyssey that would destroy her life over the coming years. Along the way, she would deal with depression, psychosis, rashes, and eventually deafness.

In each other, the two women found strong allies.

With Médecins Sans Frontières's technical assistance, the two women have filed a patent challenge to bedaquiline at the Mumbai patent office. Both want to ensure that newer, safer drugs like bedaquiline are made available to every DR TB patient and that toxic injectables are phased out.

Spelling out her reason for filing the case, Nandita told me, "My TB was not my fault. I didn't deserve it. It took me years to understand that. Our health system, government, and corporations have created a situation which has made me vulnerable to get TB . . . *just by breathing in Mumbai.* I do not agree that you need to be a perfect patient, with exact amount of sickness, living in the right country, be of the right caste or race, to get access to a lifesaving medicine."

They have challenged the patent application by Johnson & Johnson for the "salt form of bedaquiline," which does not merit patenting under India's patent law given the national health emergency.

Johnson & Johnson enjoys a monopoly on bedaquiline until 2023 and has filed a secondary patent to further extend the monopoly until 2027. If granted, Johnson & Johnson could delay the entry of generics by four additional years, evergreening its patent.

If the HIV epidemic demonstrated what was wrong with the world order and its racial implications, post-HIV plagues, TB in particular, have proved that international legal agreements like TRIPS inherently prioritize profits over black and brown lives. Dr. Mugyenyi warned that if the TRIPS laws were not seen as gross human rights violations now, future generations would look back in shock and disbelief.

A decade later, the prophecy has already proven true for TB.

Post-HIV plagues have to deal with TRIPS-Plus agreements—stronger IP laws, with stronger incentives for Big Pharma and, higher returns for companies.

In March 2018, I interviewed Dr. Soumya Swaminathan, former director general of the Indian Council of Medical Research and the current chief scientific officer for the WHO in Geneva. As she was leaving for her new job, she had one piece of advice for the

Indian government: a compulsory license for the two TB drugs: bedaquiline and delamanid.

The patent—a license given by the government to a company to have a monopoly on a drug—is much like a driving license or any other license issued by governments, who retain the right to take it away if abused.

There is precedent for it: anthrax.

Bayer held the patent, and they were charging five dollars per pill when the government needed two million pills post 9/11. The US government informed the company they'd take away the license if prices were not lowered.

Within days, the price was less than a dollar.

The Indian government, under Modi, had been unwilling to antagonize American pharmaceutical companies by issuing a compulsory license, as the Special 301 sword hangs over its head. Instead, the health ministry has "requested" Johnson & Johnson and Otsuka grant voluntary licenses to Indian manufacturers.

In a heartbeat, both companies denied the request.[14]

Meanwhile, the donation program was phased out by March 2019. Any further procurements of bedaquiline would be priced at $900 for a six-month course, while delamanid could cost each patient $1,700 for a six-month course. Patients with DR TB typically need a course of eighteen months of both drugs, which means a cost of about $7,000 per patient.

Andrew Hill, professor of molecular and clinical pharmacology at the University of Liverpool, estimates that a generic version of bedaquiline could be sold at $54–$96 and delamanid at $24–$54 for a six-month course if a generic company got a license.[15] It could cost around $150, or Rs10,946.

Dr. Farmer says the denial of new therapies to Indian patients raises several moral questions. "Anyone who has gone to Mumbai finds it hard to believe that there is no money in India. It is not a place with few resources. Why is it that India—a setting of significant resources and of an impressive industry for the manufacture of drugs and other medical products—cannot provide its own TB patients with the highest standard of care? It is grotesque that thousands of Indian patients are dying for lack of access to bedaquiline and other novel therapies. This is a moral failure."

As long as drugs are locked away behind patents, patients face the choice of being deaf or being dead.

They may not be screaming into news cameras or shutting down the FDA or the stock exchange, but TB patients are just as angry as the HIV patients of the 1990s, angry because there are no medicines. Angry because doctors are not diagnosing them properly. Angry because if and when they are diagnosed, they are treated like a disease and not like a patient. Angry at the rationing of medicines.

And above all, angry at how we have, one bad decision at a time, socially constructed a phantom plague.

CHAPTER 13

———— ◆ ————

CLINICAL DESERTS

Four months after Shreya's death, one of her treating doctors, Dr. Rohit Sarin, director of India's National Institute of Tuberculosis and Respiratory Diseases, published a study in the *Indian Journal of Tuberculosis*, saying bedaquiline was safe. "Bedaquiline is now an accepted treatment across the country. After we showed the results, India decided to make it available in all states," Dr. Sarin told me in May 2019, when I met him in his office

Dr. Sarin said it frustrated him to refuse medicines to patients, but it had to be done. "Patients die of side effects all the time. Government hospitals have so many patients that sometimes they are put on a waiting period of a year. At times, in our profession, we are not able to serve the people. In this case, one of the reasons was that the drug was not available," he said, adding that the same situation would repeat itself for delamanid.

He said the court case "was not handled in a proper way. International organizations got involved, for which there was no need. After all, we have to sort out our own problems. We cannot say that people from US will solve our problems." Here he was obliquely referring to the expert testimony provided by Dr. Jennifer Furin.

When I asked him if he was referring to Dr. Furin, he said, "I will not name anyone. When the Indian government started this drug, we did not know its safety profile. As a national program, we could not give across the board. If the patient dies as the consequence of this drug, then obviously the government cannot excuse itself. As doctors, our first job is to do no harm."

Without irony, he told me that Shreya had to be condemned to death and that *that* was doing no harm.

Dr. Sarin incorrectly said that bedaquiline's safety profile was unknown when the Indian government started the legal case. By 2016, when Shreya was fighting in Indian courts to access the drug, global scientific evidence was available, and the WHO had already issued interim guidelines recommending usage of bedaquiline.

Dr. Sarin did not want to discuss Shreya's case or the calculated injustice of it. Instead, he spoke of policy and data—from a distance, where families remain anonymized, easy to forget.

In this respect, Dr. Sarin belongs to a brutal utilitarian tradition within medicine, one that views patients as data points that are necessary for research but not as individuals whose lives must, as a priority, be saved.

Families like Shreya's can be found across India and around the world, where preventable and curable diseases are spreading in "clinical deserts" because lifesaving medicines are governed as a luxury commodity. New therapies are either not available in the Global South or rationed because of high drug prices.

Throughout medical history, creation of concentrated pockets of infectious diseases like TB, syphilis, and smallpox have resulted in them boomeranging inside clinical deserts for a while before ricocheting outward. As the gaps caused by class, caste, and race inequities widen, the global epidemic of infectious diseases, espe-cially TB, is one of the most democratic spheres of public life in India, making it a republic of suffering.

* * *

The Tuskegee Syphilis Study, like many horror stories, began with good intentions, in 1932.[1] It would go on for forty years and would set the benchmark for unethical medical research when it was stopped in 1972. It has become a globally renowned example of a government's willingness to exploit vulnerable patients for scien-tific research while setting aside genuine concern for their health and well-being.

Syphilis, an ancient sexually transmitted disease, is caused by the bacterium *Treponema pallidum.* Like all great plagues, syphilis also changed our society. Because it is sexually transmitted, like HIV today, it was also culturally associated with sinfulness, sexual deviancy, and poor hygiene.

The infection initially manifests as an ulcer in the genital area, but the sore usually goes away. It typically returns a second time, again starting with an angry rash, and is a little more serious than the first symptoms. At this point, the disease enters a latent stage—where it can remain for decades. Sometimes patients die before it comes back a third time. But when it does, it is unforgiving.

This time, it can affect many organs in the body—including the heart and the brain. Third-stage syphilis can cause large, pus-filled ulcers on the body, hair loss, blindness, mental health disor-ders, paralysis, organ failure—and death. It is disfiguring as well. The bacteria can attack the face, leaving cratered necrotic holes where a nose, a set of eyes, or a mouth ought to be.

The stigma associated with it was brutal. Patients who could buy care also bought silence—confidentiality between doctors and patients has its roots in the treatment of syphilis.

Fashion changed as well.[2]

Europe, in the 1580s, had a serious syphilitic crisis. Baldness swept the land.

For nearly two centuries, powdered wigs—called perukes—were all the rage because the king of France, Louis XIV, and the king of England, Charles II, had to start wearing wigs to avoid embarrassment. Both men likely had syphilis. The term "bigwig" comes from this.

For women, hiding syphilitic scars resulted in nose-patching, pancake makeup, and painted-on beauty spots. We also have syphilis to thank for condoms. In the mid-sixteenth century, protective sheaths made of sheep's gut became available. They were expensive and, hence, often reused—not ideal under any circumstance but an especially unfortunate choice if the idea was to protect the wearer from syphilis.[3]

In the 1920s, the Tuskegee study in Macon County, Alabama, was conceived with a clear moral purpose: to show the burden of syphilis so the national government could start an eradication program.

In the American South, syphilis was a public health crisis.

Macon County was one of the most disadvantaged places in the whole of the United States. The citizens were largely poor African American sharecroppers, during a time of full-blown racial apartheid. The county was rigidly segregated, and there was a massive health deficit in African American neighborhoods. Poor hospitals and schools meant that an overwhelming burden of disease and suffering was inflicted upon these communities. In this environment, venereal diseases were rampant.

During the first year of research, in 1932, doctors assessed the extent of the disease—conducting surveys and collecting data. At that time, 4 out of 1,000 Americans nationwide had syphilis. The outbreak within the African American community was almost double the national average: 7.2 African American men out of 1,000.

In Macon County, Alabama, it was 360 out of 1,000 African Americans. It was the hottest of the hotspots.[4]

Known officially as the Tuskegee Study of Untreated Syphilis in the Negro Male, the study began at a time when there was no known treatment for the disease. Dr. Thomas Parran was the head of the US Public Health Service's (PHS) Department of Venereal Diseases in 1929. He was approached by Oliver C. Wenger, director of the regional Venereal Disease Clinic in Mississippi, to propose a syphilis study to be sponsored by the Rosenwald Fund.

Parran had been inspired by a similar syphilis study on Nordic populations conducted in Oslo, Norway, a few years earlier. He wanted to conduct a copycat study to see how the disease affects black populations. The doctor in Oslo had withheld treatment from two thousand patients because he was convinced that the treatment available at the time was worse than the disease.

The Oslo study ended when treatment became available.

Parran wanted a similar study on black men. But it was the 1930s, and the Great Depression was ravaging America and there was little available financial support, so the PHS did not have the resources to carry out the study.[5] Later that year, Dr. Taliaferro Clark changed tack. He had just become the head of the Department of Venereal Diseases. He suggested that the project could be salvaged by conducting a prospective study on the effects of untreated syphilis on living subjects. It was initially conceived of as a six-month study. Together, Clark, Wenger, and Parran were the architects of the infamous syphilis experiments.

At the core of this experiment was a set of racially biased assumptions.

The researchers already believed that racial groups had biological differences so significant that diseases in different races followed different paths. Further, the researchers believed that African American men had a greater incidence of syphilis because of their insatiable sexual appetite.

During the 1930s, many white doctors viewed African Americans as the "syphilis-soaked race." This followed another assumption: while syphilis affected the neurological system in the white male, in African American men it did not affect the neurological system because they had smaller brains. It was presumed that the disease attacked the cardiovascular system instead.

Another damaging assumption—replicated with HIV patients in African nations and TB patients in India—was that the patients were unlikely to adhere to treatment, even though we know now that people in Macon County had been approaching physicians for treatment, in some cases multiple times.

Lastly, Dr. Clark argued that since there was no available treatment anyway and these patients were already dying, scientists might as well observe them. The operative part was to study the cadavers, postmortem, to see how the disease had progressed untreated.

Dr. Clark called it a "ready-made situation" to conduct a "study in nature." Once the study was designed, he was in a tricky situation: How do you recruit volunteers to a study that has no therapeutic benefit to the trial subject?

The men of Macon County were desperately poor, illiterate, and had almost no access to medical care. The Tuskegee Institute, now known as Tuskegee University, signed up to be the site of the study. It is a historically black university established by Booker T. Washington, American civil rights leader and educator. The university was founded for the education of freed men after the Civil War, and collaborating with it gave the study the prestige required to attract volunteers.

The PHS sent out mass mailings to black churches in Macon County. The letters promised treatment for anyone who thought they had "bad blood." The phrase in Macon County, Alabama, was elastic, a catch-all term with a number of inconsistent meanings— anemia, indigestion, and, of course, syphilis.

In addition, volunteers were promised funeral expenses, courtesy of the US government, provided they allowed the bodies to be autopsied. Knowing that it would be impossible to autopsy the body if the subject died outside the hospital, the US PHS offered $50—a small fortune for the families—to cover burial expenses. It encouraged families to bring the subjects back to the hospital if they became sick.

The men were offered food (occasionally), free transport to the treatment center, and burial insurance. Dr. Clark, who presided over the initial years of the study, directly approved the use of deception to enroll subjects.

Perhaps the most important local health-care provider linked to the project from its inception to its end was Eunice Rivers. She was an African American nurse who had trained at the Tuskegee Institute, and she was the direct link to the black community. Medical history records her either as a victim of the Jim Crow–era South or as the diabolical person who was instrumental in making sure the subjects kept returning by continuously and relentlessly lying about "treatment."

Both could be true; her own account of this episode is not known.

The Tuskegee study began by offering lower-class African Americans, who often could not afford health care, the chance to join "Miss Rivers's Lodge." From this "lodge" patients were to receive free physical examinations at Tuskegee University, free rides to and from the clinic, hot meals on examination days, and free treatment for minor ailments.

As the study became long term, Nurse Rivers became the only study staff person to work with participants for the full forty years.[6] Unlike the usual constant changing of national, regional, and on-site PHS administrators, doctors, and researchers, Rivers stayed at Tuskegee University. The fact that African Americans had almost no access to medical care resulted in an increased willingness on the part of subjects to participate in the study. For many study participants, the examination by the PHS physician was the first medical examination they had ever undergone.

Unsurprisingly, a huge number of people came forward.

The US PHS enrolled 600 black men, 399 with syphilis and 201 without, who served as a control group. The study participants received medical examinations, but none was told that he was infected with syphilis. They were either not treated or were treated with low doses of medicines insufficient to cure the disease.

From the start, the study was morally repugnant as well as scientifically invalid. It began by administrating a small dose of the accepted therapy of the day—mercury and arsenic. That decision compromised the results immediately because then it was no longer a study of *untreated* syphilis.

In order to make the men think they were being treated for their "bad blood," Dr. Wenger handed out pink-colored tablets. This "pink medicine" did not help with syphilis but did relieve minor aches and pains. It was aspirin.

The volunteers were subject to annual physical examinations, blood tests, and excruciatingly painful spinal taps. The doctors gained the "consent" of the subjects for spinal taps by depicting the diagnostic test as a "special free treatment." The lumbar puncture was for research only and had nothing to do with treatment. It is a rough procedure with potentially serious side effects.

The doctors kept the spinal tap phase for the last, worried that word about this might get around and subjects might drop out of the study. When it came time for the spinal tap, residents of Macon County received a letter from the health department:[7]

> Dear Sir:
>
> Some time ago you were given a thorough examination and since that time we hope you have gotten a great deal of treatment for bad blood. You will now be given your last chance to get a second examination. This examination is a very special one and after it is finished you will be given a special treatment if it is believed you are in a condition to stand it.

The notice ended with this sentence, in all caps:

> REMEMBER THIS IS YOUR LAST CHANCE FOR SPECIAL FREE TREATMENT. BE SURE TO MEET THE NURSE.

When America entered the Second World War, there was the danger that the study members could be drafted into the army, which would entail blood tests. If their syphilis was discovered by the army, they would be treated. The assistant surgeon general of the United States intervened on behalf of the study and provided the Selective Service Board of Macon County with the list of all those men included in the study, and they were exempted from the military draft.[8] Even so, during World War II, about fifty of the study subjects were ordered by their draft boards to undergo treatment for syphilis. The PHS requested that the draft boards exclude study subjects from the requirement for treatment.

The draft boards agreed.

By the 1940s, penicillin, a highly efficacious remedy for syphilis, had been developed. In 1943, the Henderson Act was passed, allowing venereal disease treatment to be publicly funded, and Alabama began using penicillin for treating syphilis in 1947.

While the rest of the country was cured, the trial subjects at Tuskegee were systematically denied.

To maintain this level of deception, multiple government departments and incoming heads of institutions colluded for decades. The Alabama Health Department, the US PHS, local doctors in Macon County, and the draft board worked together to make sure no one treated or recommended treatment by mistake to any of the six hundred trial subjects. The investigators also convinced *other* doctors to withhold care, and names of the trial subjects were shared, with no respect to confidentiality, to ensure a different clinic did not administer treatment by mistake.

Unlike the Oslo study, which was stopped when treatment became available, the Tuskegee study continued even after syphilis became curable. For twenty-five years after syphilis became curable, the Tuskegee study continued to deny therapy to the subjects.

In 1958, the PHS sweetened the deal by giving the men official-looking certificates of appreciation and twenty-five dollars for every year they had remained in the study. Meager as the benefits were, they had their intended effect.

It kept the men in the study.

Because the operative part of the study was the postmortem data, the trial subjects were deliberately left to degenerate as syphilis progressed—which included tumors, heart disease, paralysis, blindness, insanity, and death. With chilling candor, a physician with the US PHS said, "As I see it, we have no further interest in these patients until they die."[9]

By the end of the study in 1972, twenty-eight of the men had died as a direct result of untreated syphilis. A hundred others had died of complications related to syphilis. Forty wives of subjects of the study were infected, and nineteen children were born with congenital syphilis.

All the while, doctors wrote scholarly articles about the study, and the prevailing belief was that this was an acceptable thing to do.[10]

The Tuskegee study eventually ended after it was exposed on July 25, 1972, by an Associated Press reporter named Jean Heller. She had been tipped off by a government whistleblower, a venereal disease interviewer and investigator named Peter Buxtun.[11] In 1966, Buxtun was a twenty-seven-year-old venereal disease investigator for the US PHS, stationed in San Francisco. One day in the coffee room, Buxtun overheard a coworker talking about a syphilis patient in Alabama. Buxtun learned that the patient had been taken to a different doctor, far away from Tuskegee, where he was given a shot of penicillin and cured. The doctor, unaware of the Tuskegee study, had treated a research subject who was not supposed to be treated.

Buxtun was shocked to hear that a doctor was berated by the US PHS for "ruining one of our volunteers." He decided to investigate. He called a source at the CDC and asked for information on the Tuskegee study. A thick brown envelope soon landed on his desk.[12] He quickly learned that since 1932 the US PHS had studied untreated syphilis among four hundred African American sharecroppers. Buxtun took the reports to the nearest library. "I wanted to look up German war crimes proceedings," he told the *American Scholar* in a December 2017 interview.

Buxtun had come to America as an infant in 1937, the son of a Jewish Czech father and an Austrian mother. He knew that in the Nuremberg Trials, some German physicians were indicted for experimenting on concentration camp prisoners—seven were executed—and this had led to the modern code of research ethics.

His immediate supervisors were not pleased.

One responded, "I'll send your report up the line, but remember I have a wife and kids. Please forget my name when they ask you why you did this." Another scorned his report as "trash," insisting "the men were all volunteers."

Buxtun was summoned to Atlanta to meet William Brown, the head of the Venereal Disease Section of the US PHS, and given a "tongue-lashing" by stern-looking bureaucrats. He was expecting to be fired.

But nothing happened.

In November 1968, seven months after the assassination of Martin Luther King Jr., Buxtun wrote to Brown once again, this time pointing out the political sensitivity of the study. "The group is 100% negro. This in itself is political dynamite and subject to wild journalistic misinterpretation," Buxtun wrote.

Brown did not respond.

Instead, in 1969, a PHS committee determined that the study should continue, and this conclusion was backed by local chapters of the American Medical Association. By the early 1970s, Buxtun had left the PHS but was still living in San Francisco, where he met Edith Lederer, Associated Press correspondent, six months into her first job.

He recalled her saying, incredulous, "What? Black people? All of them black?"

Lederer asked Buxtun if he had any documentation. They hopped in his car and went straight to his apartment. "She kept looking and looking, and finally she said, 'Can I borrow this and Xerox it?'"

He said, "I wish you would."

Lederer sent the material to Jean Heller, an investigative reporter in the Washington office. Heller's article appeared on July 25, 1972, in the *New York Times* and *Washington Post* with the headline, "Syphilis Victims in U.S. Study Went Untreated for 40 Years."

It would be difficult to name a figure in the history of biomedical ethics whose actions have been more consequential than Peter Buxtun. His revelations triggered Senate hearings, a federal inquiry, a class-action lawsuit, and a lasting set of federal guidelines intended to protect trial subjects.

In 1972, the federal inquiry concluded that the Tuskegee study was "ethically unjustified"—the knowledge gained was sparse when compared with the risks the study posed for its subjects. By October 1972, the panel advised stopping the study at once.

In the summer of 1973, the study participants and families filed a class-action lawsuit. Within a year, a $10 million out-of-court settlement was reached. As part of the settlement, the US government promised to give lifetime medical benefits and burial services to all living participants.[13] The last study participant died in January 2004. The last widow receiving health benefits died in January 2009. The government-supported doctors involved in this study went on to attain great fame in their careers; although there was a lawsuit, no one was ever legally punished for what was done. Today, the Tuskegee study is one of the most enduring wounds in American medical history.

In 1976, historian James Jones interviewed John Heller, director of the Venereal Diseases Unit of the PHS from 1943 to 1948. Jones later wrote that "the men's status did not warrant ethical debate. They were subjects, not patients; clinical material, not sick people."

The Tuskegee experiment was the longest nontherapeutic experiment in medical history. A study originally designed to be conducted for six months went on for forty deadly years. PHS officials simply assumed that the study would continue until the last man had died.

The subjects were never specifically told they had syphilis or about the course of the disease. They were never consulted about what possible treatment options were available. And spinal taps were presented to them as "spinal shots"—a deceptive play on words that implied that the spinal taps had some therapeutic purpose.

The study's legacy is that it gave rise to a legally binding ethical framework for biomedical research, starting with the doctrine of "informed consent"—permission granted in full knowledge of the possible consequences, typically given by a patient to a doctor for treatment, with knowledge of the possible risks and benefits.

The study also laid out another ethical law of biomedical research—the principle of beneficence. It holds that the subjects of a medical experiment should be entitled to the expectation that some benefit will ensue from the study; the onus of it was on medical practitioners. It also laid out the guidelines stating that the most vulnerable members of a society should not be chosen as experimental subjects to the maximum extent possible. In other words, biomedical research should refrain from doing its experiments on prisoners, the mentally deficient, children, the poor, and members of disadvantaged minorities—people who can be easily misled, coerced, or intimidated.

The point of this experiment was that the subjects at Tuskegee were targeted precisely *because* they were maximally vulnerable.

On May 16, 1997, President Bill Clinton rendered the following apology to the American public. He also announced an investment to establish what would become the National Center for Bioethics in Research and Health Care at Tuskegee University.[14] At that time eight experiment survivors were alive: Charlie Pollard, Carter Howard, Fred Simmons, Frederick Moss, Sam Doner, Ernest Hendon, Herman Shaw, and George Key.

> The United States government did something that was wrong, deeply, profoundly, morally wrong. It was an outrage to our commitment to integrity and equality for all our citizens. To the survivors, to the wives and family members, the children and grandchildren, I say what you know. No power on earth can give you back the lives lost, the pain suffered, the years of internal torment and anguish. What was done cannot be undone. But we can end the silence. We can stop turning our heads away. We can look you in the eye and finally say, on behalf of the American people, what the United States government

did was shameful, and I am sorry. . . . The people who ran the study at Tuskegee diminished the stature of man by abandoning the most basic ethical precepts. They forgot their pledge to heal and repair. They had the power to heal the survivors and all the others, but they did not. Today, all we can do is apologize. But you have the power, for only you (that is, Mr. Shaw) and the others who are here, the family members who are with us in Tuskegee, only you have the power to forgive. Your presence shows that you've chosen a better path than our government did so long ago. You have not withheld the power to forgive. I hope that today and tomorrow that every American will remember this lesson and live by it.

These words of apology are now owed to millions of the world's black and brown citizens, especially in Africa and Asia, being treated with injectables that make them deaf while locking up new therapies under patents.

Clinical deserts of the twenty-first century are the moral crime of our generation.

* * *

This book began in a period of magical thinking before science, when traumatized fathers were exhuming their children to save loved ones from mysterious killers. It ends in a period of medical apartheid and science denialism that threatens to make all of us just as vulnerable to pathogens as communities were during the century when George Brown lived.

History is replete with examples of scientific progress being denied to the sick, old, poor, and vulnerable. From Tuskegee to Mumbai, in every age, societies have found racist reasons to deny salve to black and brown bodies, disproportionately affected by infectious diseases.

This is a difficult conversation to have in a world filled with strife, but it can no longer be avoided. Neither can the interplay between race and medicine be evaded. This book is an attempt to force that conversation.

Many people who look like me do not have access to basic health services and, worse yet, face trauma and humiliation when they approach medical establishments that have made a virtue out of robbing patients of their dignity. Throughout history, societies that focus their attention on the diseased state of their fellow citizens without talking about the diseased state around us—the sickness of the body politic—have failed to address the root cause that leads to pandemics: structural injustice.

Many lives are ruined by the imperfections of our global health systems. The social suffering that follows the decisions made by well-intentioned governments, philanthrocapitalists, and pharmaceutical corporations with huge blind spots have consequences.

Most global health funding comes from philanthropy. Relying on charity to solve global health is like placing a Band-Aid on a malignant tumor and expecting the patient to recover. Donations exist to affirm the hierarchies of global health and create a world in which people and countries are segregated as "high burden" and "low burden." It is a kind of public health nihilism that finds "solutions" in walling off countries, communities, and families from each other instead of making medicines affordable.

In bedaquiline's case, USAID was involved in the donation agreement between India and pharma giant Johnson & Johnson. In closed-door meetings, terms of references (still not in the public domain) were drafted to "save medicines" as patients died by the thousands. For India, depending on donations despite having sufficient manufacturing capacity is testimony to the fact that Big Pharma's takeover of the pharmacy of the world is complete.

As Nigerian novelist and poet Chinua Achebe said, "Charity . . . is the opium of the privileged."

The need of rich nations to donate stems from a deeply unsettling view of their former colonies. The West is simply unable to reimagine global health without a role for itself as the savior.

Clinical deserts—especially for curable conditions such as TB—are as much an indictment of the WHO's stewardship as they are of individual governments. The white medical establishment of the twenty-first century, deep in its marrow, continues to look at former colonies as places where diseases are to be *managed* or *controlled* without care for patients.

Then there is another rub, as pointed out by Dr. Farmer. The public health community is just as keen as corporations to skip the part that involves "caring" and instead focus on "controlling" diseases.

The deaths of Shreya and of more than 445,500 people who died from tuberculosis in 2021 are not a story limited to India or to tuberculosis. This book is an attempt to show how often social misery inflicted on black and brown nations is quantified into "targets" that truncate the stories of people like Nandita, Phumeza, and Shreya into DALYs, or "disability-adjusted life years." Cold, calculated, and self-serving statistics are used to gloss over an extortionist health system that is progressively getting worse around the world.

To reduce patients to statistics is a malevolent act in service of organizations and governments that are uncomfortable with a basic truth: it is their moral obligation, first and foremost, to protect the nation's health—its most precious asset—citizen by citizen, treating each equally and ensuring that no barriers of caste, race, gender, or pseudoscience obstruct that obligation.

Not a single shred of evidence allows the use of toxic and unsafe TB medicines when better ones are available. To deny patients like Shreya lifesaving medicines or to treat them with medicines that are making them deaf is a moral crime no different from the Tuskegee syphilis study. Rationing of bedaquiline, or any medicine, is a result of false shortage created by unfair policies. It frames health care as a zero-sum game in which there is not enough for everyone.

But there is enough for everyone.

Any shortage is curated by racist policies that do not value all lives equally. Rationing medicines, under any circumstance, has two flaws: one is economic and the other moral. Neither is justifiable.

The intellectual property laws designed to hollow out colonies centuries ago continue to do so. The patent system is a free-floating coordination between private corporations and national governments that does not prioritize the health of the nation. It selectively democratizes inequalities as well as the most expensive parts of clinical research—invariably outsourced to black and brown nations while rationing medicines in those very nations.

This callous public health strategy causes pathogens to mutate, which by extension increases the cost to control the spread of infectious diseases. A study published in the *Lancet Global Health* noted that if the business-as-usual scenario persists—that is, 31.8 million people dying from TB between 2020 and 2050—the result in economic losses will be $17.5 trillion.[15] The figure is staggering. However, the conversation about our right to health and scientific progress ought not to be had from a myopic, economic frame of reference.

Our moral flaws run deeper.

Pandemic after pandemic has tried to teach us that all the world is one family. The root of the twenty-first century's medical insecurities is the unassailable fact that minority communities rarely get to be patients. They are only research subjects in the eyes of oligopolists and power-hungry politicians.

It is a view of health as a commodity and not as a fundamental human right conferred by the state. Every person reading this, whether they are aware of it or not, is directly affected by the global patent system and the TRIPS laws. It touches every life. It is in dire need of replacement with a more responsive and democratic patent system—one that incentivizes real progress of all people, not just the Global North.

As things stand, the global trade order further reinforces poverty, economic inequity, and health deficits in minority communities around the world. Around the world, we have created a system where the rich are overtreated and overbilled, and the poor are undertreated, without compassion.

Shareholder primacy in health companies has, inch by inch, moved us away from the social reality of our era: governments in thrall of billionaires are incapable of regulating them, or their corporations, in the interest of public health. Shareholder primacy, as an ethos, is lethal in a pandemic. Decades of diverting taxes from the public sector and into private hands has led us down this inevitable path, where unconstrained capitalism is enabling unconstrained spread of diseases, even with all the miracles of modern medicine.

There is no *public* in *public health* any longer.

From penicillin to polio to the coronavirus, new therapies come to market with consistent and massive public support. Knowledge, especially scientific knowledge, does not need to be protected with patents. Knowledge is the most important input into generating future knowledge. Without Semmelweis there would be no Lister.

Besides, the argument of Big Pharma as an inventor is tiring and patently false. Owning property doesn't mean you can do whatever you want with it. For example, owning a bat doesn't mean you can hit others with it. In the same way, governments assume patent owners do not engage in anticompetitive behavior. When these assumptions are violated, governments have the right to revoke the license.

In July 2021, journalist Piergiuseppe Fortunato wrote about Big Pharma's claims about being a leading innovator:

> Despite an essentially supporting role all through the innovation process, Big Pharma can quite paradoxically claim almost exclusive intellectual-property rights (IPR) over innovations and capture notable rents on the products they manufacture. Claims to IPR via patents, copyrights and trademarks—have become one of the main means of enhancing market power, and thereby appropriating greater rents, often at the expense of wider public interests. Patent filings stood at one million in 1995. By 2011 they had more than doubled. In 2014 they reached around ten million, valued at around $15 *trillion*.[16]

Since the HIV epidemic, a lot has changed in India. Cipla is no longer headed by Dr. Hamied, and Indian generic drug makers no longer challenge patents owned by big pharmaceutical firms with the gusto of the 1990s. The Modi administration, unlike previous governments, is dealing with an increasingly ailing India using the self-destructive choice of saving patents over patients.

The combined result of these decisions is that, incrementally, India went from being the pharmacy of the world to being a contract manufacturer for the world, making affordable generics for big pharmaceutical companies that charge unacceptable prices, arrived at in secrecy. These trade policies resulted in derailing the COVID-19 response in more than one hundred developing nations, because drugs, diagnostics, protective equipment, and, most importantly, vaccines exported from India had been choked due to the deadly second wave of the coronavirus pandemic in March 2021.

In July 2021, I-MAK, a nonprofit organization of lawyers, scientists, and health experts advocating for health equity in drug development, investigated the twelve best-selling drugs in America.[17] They found that "on average, there are 131 patents filed on each medicine with 38 years of attempted patent protection blocking competition. The average price increased 71 percent, nearly nine times the rate of inflation. . . . For drugmakers, it's well worth the $25,000 investment to file and maintain a patent to delay competition. These delays are costing taxpayers hundreds of millions of dollars while further padding the pockets of drugmakers."

This is a result of capitalism without competition.

The TRIPS Agreement is fundamentally extractive, economically inefficient, and an unjustifiably racist policy, as IP and trade laws have historically been. Any corrective action must begin with scrapping the TRIPS laws. The entire underpinning of the contract is to serve not public health interests but economic ones. The latest pandemic, as with all those that came before this one, has proved that vaccine research programs (like most R&D in biopharma) are largely a result of taxpayers' investments in basic science.

The TRIPS Agreement made health care in the twenty-first century a luxury commodity instead of a right conferred to every citizen by the state. It is not simply unjust or racist. It is morally deficient—utterly devoid of compassion or a sense of justice. Any right-to-health movement must start with a full-throated call to permanently disband the TRIPS Agreement or have it renegotiated with countries in the Global South given an equal say.

Saying this is not dramatic or controversial. The moral arc of the universe does not bend toward justice. It breaks toward it.

The TRIPS law is inseparable from the racial discrimination in global health and from the egregious pricing of medicines. The pandemic has tested TRIPS and shown it to be a pack of lies sold to the developing world. The grand bargain, among the carrots the West brought out during the TRIPS negotiations, was that poorer countries will eventually be able to participate in the knowledge economy, once they become proficient in the ways of the Western world. This condescension is baked into how the West regulates knowledge and thereby the knowledge economy. The IP laws were formed when global business was concentrated in the EU. The WTO-TRIPS Agreement, the legal inheritor of nineteenth-century trade laws, serves the same purpose of loading the dice in favor of the empires. There is no doubt that the trade laws are not suitable for today's globalized world. Businesses cannot be allowed to succeed if the price of their success is paid by societies that fail. The only way black and brown patients can have more agency over their own health is by relegislating intellectual property law and radically decentering global health by placing power with the patients and not the technocrats.

Millions of TB patients die each year, unmourned. For that, will we ever be forgiven?

It is long past time to raise the bar and put a stop to this patent manipulation of controlling competition. Throughout history, tuberculosis has moved in parallel with capital *because* capital refuses to foreground collective health over personal greed. And global health cannot be trusted in the hands of the few with no interest in anything beyond greed.

The final blow to global health security has been the rise in authoritarian governments, once again a product of unconstrained capitalism and unconstrained power. In India, the rise of the Hindu supremacist movement has brought with it a tsunami of misinformation and science denialism.

The world's current predicament—with pestilence and fascism on the rise—is the pressure from the bone marrow of its economic engines to stay loyal to the culture of greed and power. From Venetian glass to bedaquiline's patent, the history of innovations has been one of collective increments. With each increment, cultural and social purposes get a back seat while personal greed becomes primary.

Incrementally, we have centralized power and concentrated a vast amount of wealth in a few hands in oligopolistic industries like Big Pharma, Big Tech, and Big Philanthropy. We can no longer tinker with language or repurpose discredited cost-effective policies to sound like a health-care plan when none of it produces the experience of accessing health care safely and humanely.

Every tragedy is also a warning. The dangers the world faces have no borders. Dr. Mugyenyi's question—"Where are the medicines, and where is the disease?"—still stands.

No amount of aid is going to save us from ever-evolving pathogens unless we fix the superstructures of global health at their structural root. TB and humans have evolved hand in hand. During the course of this relationship, the bacteria has learned from us more than we have from it.

One bad decision at a time, the global TB epidemic has been socially constructed by us—humans who are reliably small-minded, casteist, and racist every time we face a pathogen that is highly unpredictable, mutating, and thriving.

The fundamental question here is not whether the pathogen will prevail. It is whether individual decency—that encourages us to fight for the right to health and the right to dignity for the poor and vulnerable—will prevail.

There lies our salvation. No one is safe until everyone is.

ACKNOWLEDGMENTS

This book is a product of two decades of reporting on HIV and tuberculosis in India. It was conceived as an essay for *The Caravan* magazine and crystallized as I was reporting on the carnage around me, as families moved courts to access medicines.

My interest in pandemics is intricately related to my interest in politics, race, and how science interacts with social science. I hope this book will contribute to a richer understanding of the causes of the current plagues and the forces that perpetuate them.

In the seven years I worked on *Phantom Plague*, I was fortunate to be surrounded by friends, colleagues, and collaborators, without whose help I could not have completed this book. This project was born under a lucky star, nurtured by many, and I owe a debt of gratitude to everyone.

To Frank Snowden, professor of history of medicine at Yale University and Yale Open Courses, for sending me down the rabbit hole of vampire panics and for being the best teacher I never had. To the two academic homes of this book, Global Health Programs at McGill University and Nieman Foundation at Harvard University. The librarians at both universities helped me locate crucial documents and directed my attention to material I might have otherwise missed.

To Siddharth Singh, Rukun Kaul, Pratiksha Rao, Harishri Babuji, Suhasini Haider, Veena Venugopal, and Akshay and Vidya Manwani for encouraging me to write about tuberculosis (just so I stopped talking about it over dinner). To Dr. Judy Stone and Heather Stone for taking me in.

To Ali Naqvi and Elvin Lonan, who should have been here for this.

To the team behind *Phantom Plague*, who ensured the words I use are the words I mean: Kelly Falconer, agent extraordinaire, for her uncompromising belief in this project long before it was ready. To PublicAffairs, where it was edited with care by Clive Priddle and his team. To Arshu John, for meticulously fact-checking a narrative spanning centuries and continents, and to Disha Ahluwalia for a timely and last-minute assist.

To Ann Marie Lipinski and the Nieman family for what you make possible. To John and Alecia Archibald, friends and first editors. To Leena Menghaney, Tahir Amin, and other intellectual property lawyers everywhere for their unceasing belief in justice. To Mandakini Gahlot for putting up with my fascination with death and disease. To sisters everywhere.

To the survivors, caregivers, activists, doctors, and lawyers who set aside personal tragedies to fight injustice so their grief doesn't befall other families. Thank you for trusting me with your stories. It has been a privilege to witness your courage.

To readers, thank you for your time. No one should be sick because they are poor or poor because they are sick.

Inquilab Zindabad!

NOTES

Introduction

1. James Gallagher, "Analysis: Antibiotic Apocalypse," November 19, 2015, BBC News, https://www.bbc.com/news/health-21702647.

Chapter 1: The Grave of Mercy Brown

1. Michael Edward Bell, *Food for the Dead: On the Trail of New England's Vampires* (Middletown, CT: Wesleyan University Press, 2011).
2. Joe Bills, "New England's Vampire History: Legends and Hysteria," *New England Today*, October 28, 2019, https://newengland.com/today/living/new-england-history/new-england-vampire-history/.
3. Sara Davis, "The Science of Bram Stoker's Dracula," *Rosenbach*, November 3, 2017, https://rosenbach.org/blog/the-science-of-bram-stokers-dracula/.
4. Roger Luckhurst, "Why Bother Reading Bram Stoker's Dracula?" OUPblog, April 21, 2015, https://blog.oup.com/2015/04/reading-bram-stoker-dracula/.
5. Marsh's Library, "Available Online! Bram Stoker and the Haunting of Marsh's Library," accessed September 2, 2021, https://www.marshlibrary.ie/new-exhibition-bram-stoker-the-haunting-of-marshs-library/.
6. Marjie Bloy, "Cholera Comes to Britain: October 1831," Peel Web, last modified June 27, 2020, http://www.historyhome.co.uk/peel/p-health/cholera3.htm.
7. "Cholera's Seven Pandemics," CBC News, October 22, 2010, https://www.cbc.ca/news/science/cholera-s-seven-pandemics-1.758504.
8. Jessica Sutton, "Dracula and the Victorian Understanding of Disease," Sweet Goth's Vampires, March 17, 2010, http://sweetgothvampires.blogspot.com/p/normal-0-false-false-false-en-us-x-none_27.html.

9.   W. Parker Stoker, "Charlotte Matilda Blake Thornley," Bram Stoker Estate, 2018, accessed September 3, 2021, http://www.bramstokerestate.com/charlotte -matilda-blake-thornley.

10. Charlotte Stocker, "Experience of the Cholera in Ireland 1832," in *The Green Book: Writings on Irish Gothic, Supernatural and Fantastic Literature* (Dublin: Swan River Press, 2017).

11. Daniel Flynn, "'Vampire' Unearthed in Venice Plague Grave," Reuters, March 12, 2009, https://www.reuters.com/article/us-italy-vampire-idustre52b4ru200 90312.

12. Cheri Revai, *Haunted Connecticut: Ghosts and Strange Phenomena of the Constitution State* (Mechanicsburg, PA: Stackpole Books, 2006), 103.

13. Dolly Stolze, "The Vampire Slayings of 19th Century New England," *Strange Remains* (blog), November 1, 2015, https://strangeremains.com/2015/11/01/the -vampire-slayings-in-19th-century-new-england/.

14. Abigail Tucker, "The Great New England Vampire Panic," *Smithsonian Magazine*, October 2012, https://www.smithsonianmag.com/history/the-great-new -england-vampire-panic-36482878/.

Chapter 2: Dr. Ignaz Semmelweis, Savior of Mothers

1.   "Jane Seymour," Biography.com, last updated May 12, 2021, https://www.biog raphy.com/royalty/jane-seymour.

2.   Imre Zoltán, "Ignaz Semmelweis," *Encyclopedia Britannica*, last updated August 9, 2021, https://www.britannica.com/biography/Ignaz-Semmelweis.

3.   Safiya Shaikh and Daniella Caudle, "Ignaz Philipp Semmelweis (1818–1865)," Embryo Project Encyclopedia, April 6, 2017, https://embryo.asu.edu/pages /ignaz-philipp-semmelweis-1818-1865.

4.   K. Codell Carter and Barbara R. Carter, *Childbed Fever: A Scientific Biography of Ignaz Semmelweis* (Abingdon, UK: Routledge, 2017), 43–45.

5.   Miklós Kásler, "Ignaz Semmelweis, the Saviour of Mothers," *Civic Review* 14, special issue (2018): 385–410.

6.   Kerstin Michalik, "The Development of the Discourse on Infanticide in the Late Eighteenth Century and the New Legal Standardization of the Offense in the Nineteenth Century," in *Gender in Transition: Discourse and Practice in German-Speaking Europe, 1750–1830*, ed. Ulrike Gleixner and Marion W. Gray, 51–71 (Ann Arbor: University of Michigan, 2006).

7.   Kásler, "Ignaz Semmelweis, the Saviour of Mothers."

8.   Ahmet Doğan Ataman, Emine Elif Vatanoğlu-Lutz, and Gazi Yıldırım, "Medicine in Stamps-Ignaz Semmelweis and Puerperal Fever," *Journal of the Turkish German Gynecological Association* 14, no. 1 (2013): 35–39.

9.   Carter and Carter, *Childbed Fever*.

10. Carter and Carter.

11. Carter and Carter.

12. Bram Stoker, *Dracula* (Enriched Classics edition; New York: Pocket Books, 2003).

13. "Girolamo Fracastoro," Highlights from the Ruth and Lyle Sellers Medical Collection, Bridwell Library, Perkins School of Theology, SMU, accessed September 3, 2021, https://www.smu.edu/Bridwell/SpecialCollectionsandArchives /Exhibitions/Sellers2016/HistoryofMedicine/Fracastoro.

14. Russell Levine and Chris Evers, "The Slow Death of Spontaneous Generation (1668–1859)," Access Excellence, About Biotech, 1999, accessed September 3, 2021, http://webprojects.oit.ncsu.edu/project/bio183de/Black/cellintro/cellintro _reading/Spontaneous_Generation.html.

15. Julian Rubin, "Anton Van Leeuwenhoek," Juliantrubin.com, 2018, accessed September 3, 2021, https://www.juliantrubin.com/bigten/leeuwenhoek_micro scope.html.

16. Ignaz Semmelweis, *The Etiology, Concept, and Prophylaxis of Childbed Fever*, trans. by K. Codell Carter (Madison: University of Wisconsin Press, 1983).

17. Carter and Carter, *Childbed Fever.*

18. Pasteur Brewing, "Louis Pasteur Timeline: The Life of Louis Pasteur," accessed September 3, 2021, https://www.pasteurbrewing.com/louis-pasteur-timeline -the-life-of-louis-pasteur/.

19. Levine and Evers, "The Slow Death of Spontaneous Generation."

20. Agnes Ullmann, "Louis Pasteur," *Encyclopedia Britannica*, last modified September 24, 2021, https://www.britannica.com/biography/Louis-Pasteur.

21. Marea Donnelly, "Controversy Still Surrounds Louis Pasteur's 'Fantastic' Process," *Daily Telegraph*, April 20, 2017, https://www.dailytelegraph .com.au/news/controversy-still-surrounds-louis pasteurs-fantastic-process /news-story/287205a51a4a32b1bdaee1f821cc4128.

22. Ann Lamont, "Joseph Lister: Father of Modern Surgery," Answers in Genesis, March 1, 1992, https://answersingenesis.org/creation-scientists/joseph-lister -father-of-modern-surgery/.

23. "Lister, Joseph, Baron Lister of Lyme Regis (1827–1912)," Royal College of Surgeons of England, Plarr's Lives of the Fellows, April 23, 2008, https:// livesonline.rceng.ac.uk/biogs/E000500b.htm.

24. "Lister, Joseph," Royal College of Surgeons of England.

25. Wendy Moore, "'The Butchering Art' by Lindsey Fitzharris, Review—Grisly Medicine," *Guardian*, October 12, 2017, https://www.theguardian.com/books /2017/oct/12/the-butchering-art-by-lindsey-fitzharris-review.

26. Dennis Pitt and Jean Michel Aubin, "Joseph Lister: Father of Modern Surgery," *Canadian Journal of Surgery* 55, no. 5 (October 2012): E8–E9.

27. Pitt and Aubin, "Joseph Lister."

28. Richard Cavendish, "Lister Pioneers Antiseptic Surgery in Glasgow," *History Today* 65, no. 8 (August 2015), https://www.historytoday.com/archive/lister -pioneers-antiseptic-surgery-glasgow.

29. Javier Yanes, "Joseph Lister, the Man Who Sterilized Surgery," OpenMind BBVA, February 10, 2018, https://www.bbvaopenmind.com/en/science/research /joseph-lister-the-man-who-sterilized-surgery.

30. "Robert Koch," Biography.com, last updated April 16, 2019, https://www .biography.com/scientist/robert-koch.

31. "Robert Koch Biographical," NobelPrize.org, accessed September 4, 2021, https://www.nobelprize.org/prizes/medicine/1905/koch/biographical/.

32. Steve M. Blevins and Michael S. Bronze, "Robert Koch and the 'Golden Age' of Bacteriology," *International Journal of Infectious Diseases* 14, no. 9 (September 2010): e744–e751.

33. Blevins and Bronze, "Robert Koch."

34. Howard Markel, "The Day We Discovered the Cause of the 'White Death,'" PBS NewsHour, March 24, 2015, https://www.pbs.org/newshour/health /march-24-1882-robert-koch-announces-his-discovery-of-the-cause-of -tuberculosis.

35. Bacteria are transparent and colorless, which makes them invisible to the naked eye, even under the microscope. Staining with dyes allows us to see the bacterial cell and its internal structure.

36. This could qualify as a lifetime's work for any scientist, but much like his rival, Pasteur, Koch did not stop there. In 1883, a year after the dramatic TB medical conference, he made another discovery, equally influential in science to this day. This time he had discovered the agent causing cholera. Koch had diagnosed the causes of two of the most feared killers of the nineteenth century.

37. Steve Parker, *A Short History of Medicine* (New York: DK, 2019).

38. Semmelweis, *Etiology, Concept, and Prophylaxis*, 62.

39. M. Best and D. Neuhauser, "Ignaz Semmelweis and the Birth of Infection Control," *BMJ Quality and Safety* 13, no. 3 (June 2004): 233–234.

40. Shaikh and Caudle, "Ignaz Philipp Semmelweis."

41. Carter and Carter, *Childbed Fever.*

42. Carter and Carter.

Chapter 3: The Man Problem

1. Samantha Silva, "Charles Dickens Had Serious Beef with America and Its Bad Manners," Literary Hub, December 21, 2017, https://lithub.com/charles -dickens-had-serious-beef-with-america-and-its-bad-manners.

2. René Dubos and Jean Dubos, *The White Plague: Tuberculosis, Man, and Society* (New Brunswick, NJ: Rutgers University Press, 1987); Annabel Kanabus, "TB in

the United States—The Goal of Elimination," TBFacts.org, May 2020, https://tbfacts.org/tb-united-states/.

3. Barron Lerner, "New York City's Tuberculosis Control Efforts: The Historical Limitations of the 'War on Consumption,'" *American Journal of Public Health* 83, no. 5 (May 1993): 758–766.

4. "From 1892 to 1901, Biggs was a pathologist and director of the bacteriological laboratories and thereafter was general medical officer of the New York Department of Health." Wikipedia, s.v. "Hermann Biggs," last modified February 28, 2021, https://en.wikipedia.org/wiki/Hermann_Biggs.

5. Patrick J. O'Connor, "'Spitting Positively Forbidden': The Anti-Spitting Campaign, 1896–1910" (PhD dissertation, University of Montana, 2015), 4, https://scholarworks.umt.edu/cgi/viewcontent.cgi?referer=https://www.google.com/&httpsredir=1&article=5498&context=etd.

6. Shaunacy Ferro, "The Anti-Spitting Campaigns Designed to Stop the Spread of Tuberculosis," Mental Floss, November 13, 2018, https://www.mentalfloss.com/article/561579/tuberculosis-anti-spitting-campaigns.

7. O'Connor, "'Spitting Positively Forbidden.'"

8. O'Connor.

9. "History of World TB Day," Centers for Disease Control and Prevention, December 12, 2016, https://www.cdc.gov/tb/worldtbday/history.htm.

10. Theresa Machemer, "When a Women-Led Campaign Made It Illegal to Spit in Public in New York City," *Smithsonian Magazine*, February 10, 2020, https://www.smithsonianmag.com/history/19th-century-public-health-campaign-made-it-illegal-spit-public-new-york-city-180974023/.

11. "History of World TB Day."

12. O'Connor, "'Spitting Positively Forbidden,'" citing Elmer B. Borland, "JAMA 100 Years Ago: 'Municipal Regulation of the Spitting Habit,'" *Journal of the American Medical Association* 284, no. 14 (2000): 1760.

13. "The Long Victorian," *Long Victorian Prints* (blog), September 5, 2018, https://thelongvictorian.tumblr.com/post/177740538945/the-trailing-skirt-death-loves-a-shining-mark.

14. Yhe-Young Lee, "Controversies about American Women's Fashion, 1920–1945: Through the Lens of the New York Times" (PhD dissertation, Iowa State University Digital Repository, 2003), https://lib.dr.iastate.edu/cgi/viewcontent.cgi?article=1724&context=rtd.

15. Emily Mullin, "How Tuberculosis Shaped Victorian Fashion," *Smithsonian Magazine*, May 10, 2016, https://www.smithsonianmag.com/science-nature/how-tuberculosis-shaped-victorian-fashion-180959029/.

16. Steve Palace, "Why Men Started Shaving Their Beards for Health Reasons," Vintage News, November 17, 2018, https://www.thevintagenews.com/2018/11/17/beards-vs-tuberculosis/.

17. Katherine A. Foss, "How Epidemics of the Past Changed the Way Americans Lived," *Smithsonian Magazine*, April 1, 2020, https://www.smithsonianmag.com/history/how-epidemics-past-forced-americans-promote-health-ended-up-improving-life-this-country-180974555/.

18. D. Mark Anderson et al., "Was the First Public Health Campaign Successful? The Tuberculosis Movement and Its Effect on Mortality," *American Economic Journal: Applied Economics* 11, no. 2 (2019): 143–175, https://doi.org/10.3386/w23219.

19. Anthony M. Lowell, *A Half Century's Progress against Tuberculosis in New York City: 1900–1950* (New York: New York Tuberculosis and Health Association, 1952).

20. Lerner, "New York City's Tuberculosis Control Efforts."

Chapter 4: The Doctor from Southsea

1. "Arthur Conan Doyle," Encyclopædia Britannica, accessed August 31, 2021, https://www.britannica.com/biography/Arthur-Conan-Doyle.

2. Justin Brower, "Gelsemium and Sir Arthur Conan Doyle, the Self-Poisoner," *Nature's Poisons* (blog), September 18, 2014, https://naturespoisons.com/2014/08/12/gelsemium-and-arthur-conan-doyle-the-self-poisoner-gelsemine-sherlock-holmes/.

3. "Sir Arthur Conan Doyle (1859–1930) from Literary Anecdotes about 19th Century Authors Born After 1829," Our Civilisation, accessed August 31, 2021, https://www.ourcivilisation.com/smartboard/shop/anecdtes/c19/doyle.htm.

4. Sarah B. Dine, "Microbes and Mystery," *Health Affairs* 34, no. 2 (February 1, 2015): 357, https://www.healthaffairs.org/doi/full/10.1377/hlthaff.2014.1439.

5. Howard Markel, "How Dr. Arthur Conan Doyle Cracked the Case of the Tuberculosis 'Remedy,'" PBS NewsHour, May 21, 2016, https://www.pbs.org/newshour/health/how-dr-arthur-conan-doyle-cracked-the-case-of-the-tuberculosis-remedy.

6. Arthur Conan Doyle, "Dr. Koch and His Cure," Arthur Conan Doyle Encyclopedia, last modified March 26, 2017, https://www.arthur-conan-doyle.com/index.php?title=Dr._Koch_and_his_Cure.

7. Thomas Goetz's book *The Remedy: Robert Koch, Arthur Conan Doyle, and the Quest to Cure Tuberculosis* tells the fascinating story of the Conan Doyle cameo in the world of tuberculosis.

8. Arthur Conan Doyle, *The War in South Africa: Its Cause and Conduct* (London: Smith, Elder & Co., 1902).

9. Marc Barton, "Dr. Joseph Bell: The Real Life Sherlock Holmes," *Past Medical History* (blog), March 27, 2017, https://www.pastmedicalhistory.co.uk/dr-joseph-bell-the-real-life-sherlock-holmes/.

10. Barton, "Dr. Joseph Bell."

11. Charles Dickens, "Nicholas Nickleby [Excerpt]," *Academic Medicine* 80, no. 5 (May 2005): 456.

Chapter 5: Inside Building Number 10

1. Henry Sender, "An Ambani Wedding Puts the Indian Dream on Display," Nikkei Asia, March 27, 2019, https://asia.nikkei.com/Spotlight/Cover-Story /An-Ambani-wedding-puts-the-Indian-Dream-on-display.
2. "The 50,000 Square-Foot Mansion Isha Ambani's Moving Into," NDTV, December 20, 2018, https://www.ndtv.com/india-news/the-50-000-square -foot-mansion-isha-ambanis-moving-into-1965815.
3. Peehu Pardeshi et al., "Studying the Association between Structural Factors and Tuberculosis in the Resettlement Colonies in M-East Ward, Mumbai," Mumbai Metropolitan Region: Environment Improvement Society (MMR-EIS), July 2018, 10.
4. DFY partners with the Maharashtra government to run the DOTS center inside the NP Compound. DOTS, or directly observed treatment, short-course (also known as TB-DOTS), is the name given to the World Health Organization's TB control strategy. In it, a trained health-care worker or other designated individual (excluding a family member) provides the prescribed TB drugs and directly observes the patient swallow every dose.
5. Doctors at DFY, architects at IIT Bombay, and researchers from the Mumbai Metropolitan Region Environment Improvement Society, or MMR-EIS, studied three slum-redevelopment projects in Mumbai East—Natwar Parekh Compound, Lallubhai Compound, and PMG Colony.
6. Malini Krishnankutty, "For Indian Cities to Be Resilient against Disease, Housing Codes for the Poor Must Not Be Diluted," Scroll.in, July 27, 2020, https:// scroll.in/article/968388/for-indian-cities-to-be-resilient-against-disease-build ing-codes-for-the-poor-must-not-be-diluted.
7. Pardeshi et al., "Studying the Association between Structural Factors and Tuberculosis," 75.
8. Vaishnavi Chandrashekhar, "'Designed for Death': The Mumbai Housing Blocks Breeding TB," *Guardian*, April 26, 2018, https://www.theguardian.com /cities/2018/apr/26/mumbai-housing-blocks-breeding-tuberculosis-death.
9. J. F. Murray, "The Industrial Revolution and the Decline in Death Rates from Tuberculosis," *International Journal of Tuberculosis and Lung Disease* 19, no. 5 (2015): 502–503.
10. Mariam Dossal, "A Master Plan for the City: Looking at the Past," *Economic and Political Weekly* 40, no. 36 (September 2005): 3897–3900.
11. "Bombay Plague Epidemic," Wikipedia, last modified June 2, 2021, https:// en.wikipedia.org/wiki/Bombay_plague_epidemic.
12. Dossal, "A Master Plan for the City."

13. According to a *Times of India* report on April 7, 1897, cited by Sarita Mandpe in her thesis, *The Plague in Bombay (1896–98)*, colonial officials declared municipal workers to be "essential" and forbade them from leaving their workplaces.

14. Caroline E. Arnold, "The Bombay Improvement Trust, Bombay Millowners and the Debate over Housing Bombay's Millworkers, 1896–1918," *Essays in Economic & Business History* 30, no. 1 (2012): 106, https://www.ebhsoc.org/journal/index.php/ebhs/article/view/221.

15. Arnold, "The Bombay Improvement Trust."

16. Yue Zhang, "Building a Slum-Free Mumbai," Wilson Center, March 3, 2016, https://www.wilsoncenter.org/article/building-slum-free-mumbai.

17. India has a population density of 412 people per square kilometer, which ranks thirty-first in the world. In Mumbai, the population density is 21,000 people per square kilometer (54,000/square mile). "Mumbai (Greater Mumbai) City Population 2011–2021," accessed September 5, 2021, https://www.census2011.co.in/census/city/365-mumbai.html.

18. "20 Years of SRA: A Review of Slum Rehabilitation in Mumbai," *BlogURK* (blog), January 6, 2017, https://theblogurk.wordpress.com/2017/01/06/a-seminar-on-slum-rehabilitation-a-review/.

19. Zhang, "Building a Slum-Free Mumbai."

20. Vikas Kumar, "The Peculiar History and Fate of Slums in India's Big Cities," Youth Ki Awaaz, January 31, 2018, https://www.youthkiawaaz.com/2018/01/the-absurdity-of-spatial-illegality-the-case-of-mumbai-slums/.

21. World Health Organization, *Global Tuberculosis Report 2020: Executive Summary* (Geneva: WHO, 2020), https://apps.who.int/iris/bitstream/handle/10665/337538/9789240016095-eng.pdf.

22. "India TB Report 2020: National Tuberculosis Elimination Programme: Annual Report," Central TB Division, Ministry of Health and Family Welfare, March 2020, 211, https://tbcindia.gov.in/WriteReadData/l892s/India%20TB%20Report%202020.pdf.

23. XDR TB is MDR TB plus resistance to a fluoroquinolone and an injectable agent, including first-line and second-line antibiotics.

24. The term "Dalits," formerly known as Untouchables, refers to a wide range of castes considered to be outside the Hindu system of social order. Use of the term "Untouchable" and the practice of setting apart these castes were declared illegal by the Constituent Assembly of India in 1949.

25. B. R. Ambedkar, "Waiting for a Visa," ed. Frances W. Pritchett, accessed September 5, 2021, http://www.columbia.edu/itc/mealac/pritchett/00ambedkar/txt_ambedkar_waiting.html.

26. B. R. Ambedkar, *States and Minorities: What Are Their Rights and How to Secure Them in the Constitution of Free India* (C. Murphy, 1947).

27. "Bhimrao Ramji Ambedkar," Columbia Global Centers, accessed September 28, 2021, https://globalcenters.columbia.edu/content/mumbai-bhimrao-ramji-ambedkar.

28. Isabel Wilkerson, *Caste: The Origins of Our Discontents* (New York: Random House), 26.

29. W. E. B. Du Bois to B. R. Ambedkar dated July 1946, W. E. B. Du Bois Papers, Series 1. Correspondence, University of Massachusetts Amherst.

30. "Ambedkar: The Architect for Indian Constitution," Sankalp India Foundation, accessed September 5, 2021, http://www.sankalpindia.net/book/ambedkar -architect-indian-constitution.

31. The three universities conducting the study were Savitribai Phule University, Pune; Jawaharlal Nehru University, Delhi; and Indian Institute of Dalit Studies, Delhi. Anjali Marar, "Upper Caste Hindus Richest in India, Own 41% of Total Assets; ST Own 3.7%, Says Study on Wealth Distribution," *Indian Express*, February 14, 2019, https://indianexpress.com/article/india/upper-caste-hindus -richest-in-india-own-41-total-assets-says-study-on-wealth-distribution -5582984/.

32. Tommy Beer, "Top 1% of U.S. Households Hold 15 Times More Wealth Than Bottom 50% Combined," *Forbes*, October 8, 2020, https://www.forbes.com /sites/tommybeer/2020/10/08/top-1-of-us-households-hold-15-times-more -wealth-than-bottom-50-combined/?sh=5fccae1b5179.

33. Naveen Bharathi, Deepak Malghan, and Andaleeb Rahman, *Isolated by Caste: Neighbourhood-Scale Residential Segregation in Indian Metros* (Ithaca, NY: Dyson School of Applied Economics and Management Cornell University, May 2018), https://dyson.cornell.edu/wp-content/uploads/sites/5/2019/02/Cornell -Dyson-wp1808.pdf.

34. Bharathi, Malghan, and Rahman, *Isolated by Caste*.

35. According to the WHO, patients with drug-susceptible TB (where the bacteria is susceptible to antibiotics) have an 85 percent success rate when put on treatment. The treatment success rate for patients with DR TB falls to 57 percent globally. The treatment success rate for XDR TB falls further, to 30 percent. At this point, the patient stops responding to most antibiotics known to modern medicine.

36. Pardeshi et al., "Studying the Association between Structural Factors and Tuberculosis," 54, 76.

37. Pardeshi et al.

38. Pardeshi et al.

Chapter 6: Antibiotic Apocalypse, on the Move

1. Identities of the family featured in this story have been withheld.

2. Mishra Gyanshankar and Mulani Jasmin, "Tuberculosis Prescription Practices in Private and Public Sector in India," *National Journal of Integrated Research in Medicine* 4, no. 2 (2013): 71–78.

3. "World TB Day: A Conversation with a TB Warrior from India," Longitude Team interviewing Dr. Zarir F. Udwadia, March 24, 2017, https://www .drzarirudwadia.com/world-tb-day-conversation-tb-warrior-india/.

4. Z. F. Udwadia, L. M. Pinto, and M. W. Uplekar, "Tuberculosis Management by Private Practitioners in Mumbai, India: Has Anything Changed in Two Decades?," *PLoS ONE* 5, no. 8 (2010): e12023.

5. A. Kwan et al., "Variations in the Quality of Tuberculosis Care in Urban India: A Cross-sectional, Standardized Patient Study in Two Cities," *PLoS Medicine* 15, no. 9 (2018): e1002653.

6. C. T. Sreeramareddy et al., "Delays in Diagnosis and Treatment of Pulmonary Tuberculosis in India: A Systematic Review," *International Journal of Tuberculosis and Lung Disease* 18, no. 3 (2014): 255–266, https://doi.org/10.5588/ijtld .13.0585.

7. Ole Benedictow, "The Black Death: The Greatest Catastrophe Ever," *History Today*, March 3, 2005, https://www.historytoday.com/archive/black-death -greatest-catastrophe-ever.

8. *Guidelines for the Use of Delamanid in the Treatment of Drug Resistant TB in India*, Revised National Tuberculosis Control Programme, Central TB Division, Directorate General of Health Services, Ministry of Health and Family Welfare (New Delhi: World Health Organization, 2018), 8, https://tbcindia.gov.in /showfile.php?lid=3343.

9. "Country Updates," DR-TB STAT, last updated March 2020, http://drtb-stat .org/country-updates/.

Chapter 7: Shreya

1. The hearings in Indian courts are not recorded. Her parents have retreated from the public eye and prefer not to engage with the media. My reporting is based on interviews I did in 2016 with the family, her doctors, her lawyers, and activists, as well as transcripts from court documents—all of which capture the story in minute detail, to its miserable end.

2. Vidya Krishnan, "My Daughter Is Dying, Save Her," *Hindu*, January 9, 2017, https://www.thehindu.com/sci-tech/health/%E2%80%98My-daughter-is -dying-save-her%E2%80%99/article17014224.ece.

3. Amrit Dhillon, "Politics and Protocol Leave Indian Teen's Life in the Balance Pending TB Drug Ruling," *Guardian*, January 13, 2017, https://www.theguard ian.com/global-development/2017/jan/13/politics-protocol-indian-teen-life -in-balance-tb-drug-ruling-shreya-tripathi-tuberculosis-bedaquiline.

4. South Africa—which has a TB burden second only to India's—in 2018 became the first country to make bedaquiline available for free from its government hospitals.

5. Jennifer Furin, "TB Killed Shreya Tripathi, but Her Death Could Have Been Avoided," Wire, March 30, 2019, https://thewire.in/health/multi-drug -resistant-tb-bedaquiline-deaths.

6.   Mark Hay, "You Can't Patent Toast," My Recipes, February 13, 2018, https://www.myrecipes.com/extracrispy/you-cant-patent-toast.

7.   Malcolm Daniel, "William Henry Fox Talbot (1800–1877) and the Invention of Photography," Heilbrunn Timeline of Art History, Met Museum, October 2004, https://www.metmuseum.org/toah/hd/tlbt/hd_tlbt.htm.

8.   "Thomas Edison Patents the Kinetograph," History, February 9, 2010, last modified August 28, 2020, https://www.history.com/this-day-in-history/edison-patents-the-kinetograph.

9.   Ove Granstrand, "Innovation and Intellectual Property," Background Paper to the Concluding Roundtable Discussion on IPR at the DRUID Summer Conference, Copenhagen, June 12–14, 2003, DOI:10.1093/oxfordhb/9780199286805.003.0010.

10. Joe Mullin, "Infamous 'Podcast Patent' Heads to Trial," ArsTechnica, May 9, 2014, https://arstechnica.com/tech-policy/2014/09/jim-logan-says-he-invented-podcasts-next-week-a-jury-decides/.

11. "Episode 462: When Patents Hit the Podcast," *Planet Money*, May 31, 2013, podcast, https://www.npr.org/transcripts/187374157.

12. "Staff Attorney Daniel Nazer Becomes New 'Mark Cuban Chair to Eliminate Stupid Patents,'" Electronic Frontier Foundation, March 10, 2014, https://www.eff.org/press/releases/staff-attorney-daniel-nazer-becomes-new-mark-cuban-chair-eliminate-stupid-patents.

13. Sherrington Ailsa, "How Lush Is Elevating the Retail Experience through Ethical Technology," Next Web, May 3, 2019, https://thenextweb.com/news/lush-retail-ethical-tech.

14. Timothy B. Lee, "A Patent Lie," *New York Times*, June 9, 2007, https://www.nytimes.com/2007/06/09/opinion/09lee.html.

15. Kavaljit Singh, "War Profiteering: Bayer, Anthrax and International Trade," Corpwatch, November 5, 2001, https://corpwatch.org/article/war-profiteering-bayer-anthrax-and-international-trade.

16. The medical aid organization MSF invested in additional trials of its own. Johnson & Johnson collected data of patients on treatment by the national programs of India and South Africa.

17. "Grounds for Opposing Patent Application for Bedaquiline Formulation in India," MSF Access Campaign, February 2019, https://msfaccess.org/sites/default/files/2019-02/BDQ%20Opposition_Briefing%20Document_India_Fab2019_ENG.pdf.

18. "Grounds for Opposing Patent Application for Bedaquiline Formulation in India."

19. *A Review of the Bedaquiline Patent Landscape: A Scoping Report*, UNITAID Secretariat, World Health Organization, January 2014, http://unitaid.org/assets/TMC_207_Patent_Landscape.pdf.

20. James Hamblin, "Why Doctors Without Borders Refused a Million Free Vaccines," *Atlantic*, October 14, 2016, https://www.theatlantic.com/health /archive/2016/10/doctors-with-borders/503786/.

21. Jason Cone, "There Is No Such Thing as 'Free' Vaccines: Why We Rejected Pfizer's Donation Offer of Pneumonia Vaccines," *MSF Access Campaign* (blog), October 10, 2016, https://msf-access.medium.com/there-is-no-such-thing-as-free-vaccines -why-we-rejected-pfizers-donation-offer-of-pneumonia-6a79c9d9f32f.

22. Rohit Sarin et al., "Initial Experience of Bedaquiline Implementation under the National TB Programme at NITRD, Delhi, India," *Indian Journal of Tuberculosis* 66, no. 1 (2019): 209–213, https://doi.org/10.1016/j.ijtb.2019.02.009.

Chapter 8: The Cursed Duet

1. "Living with HIV—Dying of TB: CDC Accelerates TB Prevention for People Living with HIV," Centers for Disease Control and Prevention, last modified September 26, 2019, https://www.cdc.gov/globalhivtb/who-we-are/features /tbpreventivetherapy.html.

2. John Leland, "Twilight of a Difficult Man: Larry Kramer and the Birth of AIDS Activism," *New York Times*, May 19, 2017, https://www.nytimes.com/2017 /05/19/nyregion/larry-kramer-and-the-birth-of-aids-activism.html.

3. Leland, "Twilight of a Difficult Man."

4. Michael Shnayerson, "Kramer vs. Kramer," *Vanity Fair*, April 3, 2014, https:// www.vanityfair.com/news/1992/10/larry-kramer.

5. James W. Curran and Harold W. Jaffe, "AIDS: The Early Years and CDC's Response," Centers for Disease Control and Prevention, October 7, 2011, https://www.cdc.gov/mmwr/preview/mmwrhtml/su6004a11.htm.

6. Warren J. Blumenfeld, "God and Natural Disasters: It's the Gays' Fault?," *Huffington Post*, February 2, 2016, https://www.huffpost.com/entry/god-and -natural-disasters-its-the-gays-fault_b_2068817.

7. William F. Buckley Jr., "Crucial Steps in Combating the AIDS Epidemic: Iden-tify All the Carriers," *New York Times*, March 18, 1986, https://archive.nytimes .com/www.nytimes.com/books/00/07/16/specials/buckley-aids.html.

8. "About the Ryan White HIV/AIDS Program," Health Resources and Ser-vices Administration, last modified December 2020, https://hab.hrsa.gov /about-ryan-white-hivaids-program/about-ryan-white-hivaids-program.

9. Olivia B. Waxman, "Freddie Mercury Didn't Want to Be a 'Poster Boy' for AIDS—but He and Other Celebrities Played a Key Role in Its History," *Time*, November 5, 2018, http://time.com/5440824/freddie-mercury-celebrity-aids-awareness/.

10. Mary Elizabeth Williams, "Here's What Magic Johnson's Done, Donald Ster-ling," *Salon*, May 13, 2014, https://www.salon.com/2014/05/13/heres_what _magic_johnsons_done_donald_sterling/.

11. "Larry Kramer on the Beginning of ACT-UP," Stonewall Archive material of
     Larry Kramer on the beginnings of ACT-UP, gogaydvd, video, 3:42, April 10,
     2007, https://www.youtube.com/watch?v=ett_Rz_eNqA.

12. Douglas Crimp, "Before Occupy: How AIDS Activists Seized Control of
     the FDA in 1988," *Atlantic*, December 6, 2011, https://www.theatlantic
     .com/health/archive/2011/12/before-occupy-how-aids-activists-seized
     -control-of-the-fda-in-1988/249302/.

13. "Act Up Demonstrations on Wall Street," NYC LGBT Historic Sites Proj-
     ect, accessed September 5, 2021, https://www.nyclgbtsites.org/site/act-up
     -demonstration-at-the-new-york-stock-exchange/.

14. David Handelman, "Act Up in Anger," *Rolling Stone*, March 8, 1990, https://
     www.rollingstone.com/culture/culture-news/aids-activism-larry-kramer
     -act-up-fauci-241225/.

15. Jason Deparle, "111 Held in St. Patrick's AIDS Protest," *New York Times*,
     December 11, 1989, https://www.nytimes.com/1989/12/11/nyregion/111-held
     -in-st-patrick-s-aids-protest.html.

16. "Day of Desperation Synopsis," Act Up Historical Archive, accessed September
     5, 2021, https://actupny.org/diva/synDesperation.html.

17. Daniel Lewis, "Larry Kramer, Playwright and Outspoken AIDS Activist, Dies
     at 84," *New York Times*, May 27, 2020, https://www.nytimes.com/2020/05/27
     /us/larry-kramer-dead.html.

Chapter 9: Wretched of the Earth

1. Martin J. Vincent et al., "Chloroquine Is a Potent Inhibitor of SARS Coro-
    navirus Infection and Spread," *Virology Journal* 2, no. 69 (2005), https://doi
    .org/10.1186/1743-422X-2-69.

2. "Global HIV & AIDS Statistics—Fact Sheet," UNAIDS, accessed September
    7, 2021, https://www.unaids.org/en/resources/fact-sheet.

3. "Fact Sheet on Tuberculosis (TB)," WHO TB Department, accessed September
    7, 2021, https://www.who.int/3by5/TBfactsheet.pdf.

4. "The Pharmaceutical Industry and Global Health: Facts and Figures 2017,"
    International Federation of Pharmaceutical Manufacturers and Associations,
    2017, https://www.ifpma.org/wp-content/uploads/2017/02/IFPMA-Facts-And
    -Figures-2017.pdf.

5. "The Durban Declaration," *Nature* 406, no. 15–16 (2000), https://doi.org/10
    .1038/35017662.

6. Peter Mugyenyi, *Genocide by Denial: How Profiteering from HIV/AIDS Killed
    Millions* (Kampala, Uganda: Fountain, 2008).

7. "Commission World Health Organisation and Joint United Nations Pro-
    gramme on HIV/AIDS Take a United Stand against Killer Diseases,"

European Commission, September 28, 2000, https://ec.europa.eu/commission /presscorner/detail/en/IP_00_1072.

8.   Amy Roeder, "The Cost of South Africa's Misguided AIDS Policies," *Harvard Public Health*, spring 2009, https://www.hsph.harvard.edu/news/magazine/spr 09aids/.

9.   Sarah Boseley, "Mbeki AIDS Denial 'Caused 300,000 Deaths,'" *Guardian*, November 26, 2008, https://www.theguardian.com/world/2008/nov/26/aids -south-africa.

10.   Michael Specter, "The Denialists," *New Yorker*, March 5, 2007, https://www .newyorker.com/magazine/2007/03/12/the-denialists.

11.   "South Africa," UNAIDS, accessed July 12, 2021, www.unaids.org/en/regions countries/countries/southafrica.

12.   Kate Wilkinson, "Yes, South Africa Has the World's Largest Antiretroviral Therapy Programme," Africa Check, November 30, 2015, https://africacheck .org/reports/yes-south-africa-has-the-worlds-largest-antiretroviral-therapy -programme/.

13.   An Indian pharmaceutical company, Aurobindo Pharma Ltd., had already won the tender for supplying this drug in June 2014—a month after the Modi government had come to power. However, for three months, the ministry failed to issue a notification of awards through its procurement agent, RITES Ltd. As this document was stuck somewhere in the labyrinth of Indian bureaucracy, the company could not start manufacturing the drug.

14.   Neetu Chandra Sharma, "Health Ministry Struggles to Afford Overseas Experts after Centre's Foreign NGO Crackdown," *India Today*, April 21, 2016, www.indiatoday.in/mail-today/story/health-gasps-as-union-health-ministry -struggles-to-keep-foreign-funded-consultants-319052-2016-04-21.

15.   Richard Hurley, "HIV/AIDS: Complacency Risks Reversing Progress on Ending Epidemic, Conference Hears," *BMJ*, July 25, 2018, https://www.bmj.com /content/362/bmj.k3241.

16.   "Fire in the Blood," Transcription, 2013, https://www.mediaed.org/transcripts /Fire-In-The-Blood-Transcript.pdf.

17.   Katherine Eban, "How an Indian Tycoon Fought Big Pharma to Sell AIDS Drugs for $1 a Day," Quartz India, July 15, 2019, https://qz.com/india/1666032 /how-indian-pharma-giant-cipla-made-aids-drugs-affordable/.

18.   "Dr. Y.K. Hamied's Speech at the European Commission (28 Sept 2000)," speech delivered in Brussels on September 28, 2000, Cipla, video, 4:54, January 6, 2017, https://www.youtube.com/watch?v=NK7GDpYjGXM.

19.   Sarah Boseley, "Yusuf Hamied, Generic Drugs Boss," *Guardian*, February 18, 2003, https://www.theguardian.com/world/2003/feb/18/aids.sarahboseley13.

20.   "Cipla Dismisses Glaxo 'Piracy' Allegation," Reuters via Rediff.com, March 13, 2001, https://www.rediff.com/money/2001/mar/13cipla.htm.

21. Sunil K. Sahu, "Globalization, WTO, and the Indian Pharmaceutical Industry," *Asian Affairs: An American Review* 41, no. 4 (2014): 172–202, https://doi.org/10.1080/00927678.2014.970930.

22. Ellen 't Hoen, *Private Patents and Public Health: Changing Intellectual Property Rules for Access to Medicines* (Amsterdam: Health Action International, 2016), 7.

23. "Fire in the Blood," Transcription, 2013.

24. "Patent Situation of HIV/AIDS-Related Drugs in 80 Countries," UNAIDS and WHO, January 2000, https://www.who.int/3by5/en/patentshivdrugs.pdf.

25. Mugyenyi, *Genocide by Denial*.

Chapter 10: Patents versus Patients

1. Megan Twohey and Nicholas Kulish, "Bill Gates, the Virus and the Quest to Vaccinate the World," *New York Times*, November 23, 2020, https://www.nytimes.com/2020/11/23/world/bill-gates-vaccine-coronavirus.html.

2. Alexander Zaitchik, "How Bill Gates Impeded Global Access to COVID Vaccines," *New Republic*, April 12, 2021, https://newrepublic.com/article/162000/bill-gates-impeded-global-access-covid-vaccines.

3. Twohey and Kulish, "Bill Gates."

4. Dan Jones, "Becoming a Victorian," *Spectator*, March 20, 2010, https://www.spectator.co.uk/article/becoming-a-victorian.

5. Robert Blake and Wm. Roger Louis, *Churchill* (New York: Oxford University Press, 1993), 464.

6. Richard Toye, *Churchill's Empire: The World That Made Him and the World He Made* (New York: St. Martin's Griffin, 2010), xii.

7. Elliott Roosevelt, *As He Saw It* (New York: Duell, Sloan and Pearce, 1946), 37.

8. Supriti Malhotra, "With Shashi Tharoor's 'An Era of Darkness,' the British Empire's Indictment Continues," TheSeer, May 10, 2020, https://theseer.in/with-shashi-tharoors-an-era-of-darkness-the-british-empires-indictment-continues/.

9. Yide Ma and Haoran Zhang, "Development of the Sharing Economy in China: Challenges and Lessons," in *Innovation, Economic Development, and Intellectual Property in India and China*, ed. K. C. Liu and U. Racherla (Singapore: Springer, 2019), https://doi.org/10.1007/978-981-13-8102-7_20.

10. Carolyn Deere, *The Implementation Game: The TRIPS Agreement and the Global Politics of Intellectual Property Reform in Developing Countries* (Oxford: Oxford University Press, 2009), 11.

11. Deere, *The Implementation Game*.

12. Valbona Muzaka, *The Politics of Intellectual Property Rights and Access to Medicines* (New York: Palgrave Macmillan, 2011).

13. Deere's book states that the European Commission was "sometimes sending in negotiators to conclude a bilateral agreement on intellectual property with

a developing country after U.S. negotiators had brought that country to the negotiating table using the 301 process." Deere, *The Implementation Game*, 18.

14. Deere, *The Implementation Game*, 23.
15. Deere, 23.
16. Hoen, *Private Patents and Public Health.*
17. "Doha Declaration on TRIPS and Public Health," World Health Organization, November 14, 2001, https://www.who.int/medicines/areas/policy/trips health.pdf.
18. Pat Sidley, "Drug Companies Sue South African Government over Generics," *BMJ*, February 24, 2001, https://doi.org/10.1136/bmj.322.7284.447.

Chapter 11: The Business of Dying

1. R. Prasad, "Nandita Vekatesan's Story of Recovery," *Hindu*, December 10, 2016, https://www.thehindu.com/sci-tech/health/Nandita-Venkatesan's-story-of-recovery/article16784924.ece.
2. Tanvi Dubey, "Tuberculosis Took Away 22 kg and Most of Her Hearing, but Nandita Continues to Dance to the Music of Life," YourStory, January 4, 2016, https://yourstory.com/2016/01/nandita-venkatesan.
3. "From Sound to Silence—Lessons from My Journey into Hearing Loss | Nandita Venkatesan | TEDxJECRC," TEDx talks, video, 28:48, June 21, 2017, https://www.youtube.com/watch?v=mdrYZ3mXxtI.

Chapter 12: The Phantom Plague and the Missing Millions

1. Zarir F. Udwadia et al., "Totally Drug-Resistant Tuberculosis in India," *Clinical Infectious Diseases* 54, no. 4 (2012): 579–581, https://doi.org/10.1093/cid/cir889.
2. C. Sohini, "A Tale of Two Doctors and India's History of Hiding Its Diseases," Wire, November 17, 2017, https://thewire.in/health/tale-two-doctors -indias-history-hiding-diseases.
3. *Totally Drug Resistant TB: A WHO Consultation on the Diagnostic Definition and Treatment Options* (Geneva: WHO/HQ, March 21–22, 2012), https://www .who.int/tb/challenges/xdr/Report_Meeting_totallydrugresistantTB_032012 .pdf.
4. Geeta Anand, "Battling Drug-Resistant TB, and the Indian Government," *New York Times*, September 2, 2016, https://www.nytimes.com/2016/09/03/world /asia/zarir-udwadia-india-tuberculosis-tb.html.
5. Benjamin Daniels et al., "Lessons on the Quality of Tuberculosis Diagnosis from Standardized Patients in China, India, Kenya, and South Africa," *Journal of Clinical Tuberculosis and Other Mycobacterial Diseases* 16 (2019): 100109, https://doi.org/10.1016/j.jctube.2019.100109.
6. Daniels et al., "Lessons on the Quality of Tuberculosis Diagnosis."

7.   Special Correspondent, "India Under-reported TB for 15 Years: WHO," *Hindu*, October 14, 2016, https://www.thehindu.com/sci-tech/health/India-under -reported-TB-for-15-years-WHO/article16070274.ece.

8.   The WHO revised the global TB burden from 6.1 million cases in 2015 to 10.4 million in 2016.

9.   Annabel Kanabus, "DOTS & DOTS-Plus—Failed Global Plans," TBFacts. org, last modified September 2020, https://tbfacts.org/dots-tb/.

10.   Kanabus, "DOTS & DOTS-Plus."

11.   Helen Cox and Jennifer Furin, "The Incalculable Costs of Tuberculosis," *Lancet Global Health* 9, no. 10 (2021): E1337–E1338, https://doi.org/10.1016 /S2214-109X(21)00345-4.

12.   Cox and Furin, "The Incalculable Costs."

13.   "TB Survivor Nandita Venkatesan at UNGA: 'I Can't Hear You, but I'll Make Sure You Hear Me Loud and Clear,'" *India West*, October 4, 2018.

14.   As things stand, Otsuka has signed a distribution agreement with Mylan Pharmaceuticals, the Indian subsidiary of an American pharmaceutical firm. Johnson & Johnson has yet to sign a voluntary license with an Indian drug maker to make a generic version of the medicine.

15.   D. Gotham et al., "Estimated Generic Prices for Novel Treatments for Drug-Resistant Tuberculosis," *Journal of Antimicrobial Chemotherapy* 72, no. 4 (2017): 1243–1252, https://doi.org/10.1093/jac/dkw522.

Chapter 13: Clinical Deserts

1.   "The US Public Health Service Syphilis Study at Tuskegee: Tuskegee Timeline," Centers for Disease Control and Prevention, last updated April 22, 2021, https://www.cdc.gov/tuskegee/timeline.htm.

2.   Sarah Dunant, "Syphilis, Sex and Fear: How the French Disease Conquered the World," *Guardian*, May 17, 2013, https://www.theguardian.com/books /2013/may/17/syphilis-sex-fear-borgias.

3.   Ruth Goodman, "The Victorian Condom," *Atlantic*, December 15, 2014, https:// www.theatlantic.com/magazine/archive/2014/12/vsbe-condoms/382245/.

4.   "21. The Tuskegee Experiment," lecture by Dr. Frank Snowden on the Tuskegee Experiment on Syphilis Carried Out in Macon County, Alabama, from 1932 to 1972, YaleCourses, video, 51:06, March 17, 2011, https://www.youtube.com /watch?v=3KL7lcWMkz0&ab_channel=YaleCourses.

5.   "The Tuskegee Syphilis Study," *Dartmouth Undergraduate Journal of Science*, November 12, 2008, https://sites.dartmouth.edu/dujs/2008/11/12/a-wake-up -call-for-bioethics-examining-the-tuskegee-syphilis-study/.

6.   George Sarka, "The Role of the United States Public Health Service in the Control of Syphilis during the Early 20th Century" (DPH dissertation, UCLA, 2013), 104, https://escholarship.org/content/qt4qv4b0hj/qt4qv4b0hj.pdf.

7. Sharlene Nagy Hesse-Biber and Patricia Leavy, *The Practice of Qualitative Research* (Los Angeles: SAGE, 2011), chap. 4.

8. Frank Snowden, "The Tuskegee Syphilis Experiments: A Forty-Year Mask of Shame," Brewminate, February 14, 2017, https://brewminate.com/the-tuskegee-syphilis-experiments-a-forty-year-mark-of-shame/.

9. Borgna Brunner, "The Tuskegee Syphilis Experiment," Infoplease, last modified January 25, 2021, https://www.infoplease.com/history/black-history/the-tuskegee-syphilis-experiment.

10. John Parascandola, *Sex, Sin and Science: A History of Syphilis in America* (London: Greenwood, 2018), 83.

11. Derek Kerr and Maria Rivero, "Whistle Blower Peter Buxtun and the Tuskegee Syphilis Study," Government Accountability Project, April 30, 2014, https://whistleblower.org/uncategorized/whistleblower-peter-buxtun-and-the-tuskegee-syphilis-study/.

12. Carl Elliot, "The Tuskegee Truth Teller," *American Scholar*, December 4, 2017, https://theamericanscholar.org/tuskegee-truth-teller/#.XPJ8M9P7SfQ.

13. "Tuskegee Timeline," Centers for Disease Control and Prevention.

14. "Tuskegee Timeline," Centers for Disease Control and Prevention.

15. S. Silva et al., "Economic Impact of Tuberculosis Mortality in 120 Countries and the Cost of Not Achieving the Sustainable Development Goals Tuberculosis Targets: A Full-Income Analysis," *Lancet Global Health* 9, no. 10 (2021): E1372–E1379, https://doi.org/10.1016/S2214-109X(21)00299-0.

16. Piergiuseppe Fortunato, "Fighting COVID-19 Requires Fewer Patents and More State," Social Europe, July 20, 2021, https://socialeurope.eu/fighting-covid-19-requires-fewer-patents-and-more-state.

17. Priti Krishtel, "4 Recommendations to Guide the FDA in Its Analysis of the U.S. Patent System," I-MAK, July 30, 2021, https://i-makglobal.medium.com/4-recommendations-to-guide-the-fda-in-its-analysis-of-the-u-s-patent-system-6f212b6d9d82.

APPENDIX

Table 1. Public Investments in Bedaquiline's Development[1]

No.	Study name	Description	Sponsor
1	ACTG A5343 NCT02583048	To evaluate the safety of bedaquiline when coadministered with novel TB drug, delamanid, for the treatment of MDR TB.	NIAID
2	STREAM stage II NCT02409290	To evaluate whether bedaquiline can shorten treatment to six months or replace the injectable agent in the standardized nine- to twelve-month regimen for the treatment of MDR TB. *This study will serve as Janssen's phase III trial for bedaquiline, a condition of the accelerated approval granted by the FDA in 2012.	USAID

(*continued*)

Table 1. Public Investments in Bedaquiline's Development (*continued*)

No.	Study name	Description	Sponsor
3	endTB NCT02754765	To evaluate six-month regimens composed of different combinations of bedaquiline, delamanid, linezolid, pyrazinamide, clofazimine, and moxifloxacin or levofloxacin for the treatment of MDR TB.	Unitaid
4	NEXT NCT02454205	To evaluate six to nine months of linezolid, bedaquiline, levofloxacin, pyrazinamide, and ethionamide/high dose isoniazid for the treatment of MDR TB.	University of Cape Town
5	TB-PRACTECAL NCT02589782	To evaluate six-month regimens containing bedaquiline, pretomanid, and linezolid with and without moxifloxacin or clofazimine for the treatment of MDR TB.	MSF
6	NC-003 NCT01691534	To evaluate the bacteriacidal activity of bedaquiline combined with pretomanid and pyrazinamide at two weeks. The results of NC-003 informed regimen selection for NC-005 (listed next).	TB Alliance*
7	NC-005 NCT02193776	To evaluate the early efficacy and safety of bedaquiline, pretomanid, and pyrazinamide, with and without moxifloxacin, over two months of treatment. The results of NC-005 informed regimen selection for SimpliciTB (listed next).	TB Alliance*

(*continued*)

Table 1. Public Investments in Bedaquiline's Development (*continued*)

No.	Study name	Description	Sponsor
8	SimpliciTB NCT03338621	To evaluate four months of bedaquiline, pretomanid, moxifloxacin, and pyrazinamide for the treatment of DS TB.	TB Alliance*
9	NIX-TB NCT02333799	To evaluate six to nine months of bedaquiline, pretomanid, and linezolid for the treatment of XDR TB and pre-XDR TB.	TB Alliance*
10	ZeNix NCT03086486	To evaluate six to nine months of bedaquiline and pretomanid when given with different doses and durations of linezolid for the treatment of XDR TB, pre-XDR TB, or treatment of intolerant or nonresponsive MDR TB.	TB Alliance*
11	TRUNCATE TB NCT03474198	To evaluate two-month regimens composed of first-line medicines in combination with new and repurposed second-line medicines for the treatment of DS TB.	University College London
12	ACTG A5267 NCT00992069	To evaluate the safety and effect of bedaquiline when given with efavirenz to healthy volunteers.	NIAID
13	Janssen C211 NCT02354014	To determine the dose and safety of bedaquiline in children with MDR TB, excluding those living with HIV.	Unitaid

(*continued*)

Table 1. Public Investments in Bedaquiline's Development (*continued*)

No.	Study name	Description	Sponsor
		A Unitaid-funded pediatric TB project (the STEP-TB project) contributed $1 million to this study, the conduct of which is a condition of the approval granted to Janssen by the EMA in 2014.	
14	IMPAACT P1108 NCT02906007	To determine the dose and safety of bedaquiline in children with MDR TB, including those living with HIV.	NIAID

NIAID: United States National Institutes of Allergy and Infectious Diseases
* The TB Alliance funds its trials with contributions from public and philanthropic donors.
[1] Lindsay McKenna, *The Price of Bedaquiline*, Treatment Action Group, 2018, http://www.treatmentactiongroup.org/sites/default/files/reality_check _bedaquiline_10_16_18.pdf.

Table 2. Incentives from Which Janssen Has Benefited[1]

Incentive	Description
US Orphan Drug Tax Credit	A USG tax credit worth up to 50 percent of annual R&D expenditures and other qualifying costs. This credit can be applied from the time of orphan drug designation up to approval. Bedaquiline was granted an orphan drug designation in January 2005 and approved by the FDA in December 2012. Janssen also received a tax credit for the cost of its global donation program (60,000 six-month courses of bedaquiline).

(*continued*)

Table 2. Incentives from Which Janssen Has Benefited (*continued*)

Incentive	Description
FDA marketing application fee exemption	Sponsors of drugs awarded orphan drug designation are exempt from paying marketing application fees under the US Prescription Drug User Fee Act (PDUFA): $1,841,500 in 2012.
US Tropical Disease Priority Review Voucher (PRV): PRV 204384	Sponsors that successfully register a drug for a tropical disease with the FDA are awarded a PRV, which can be used to expedite FDA review of another product or sold to another sponsor. PRVs have sold for $67–350 million. Janssen used its PRV to expedite FDA review of guselkumab (Tremfya), a blockbuster psoriasis drug that sells at nearly US$60,000 per patient per year in the US and is estimated to yield US$3.49 billion in sales by 2024. The PRV afforded Janssen a four-month jump on the market.
Additional marketing exclusivity in the US and Europe	Sponsors that successfully register an orphan drug with the FDA are awarded seven years of marketing exclusivity from the time of approval in the US (December 2012 through December 2019 in the case of bedaquiline). Sponsors that successfully register an orphan drug with the EMA are awarded ten years of marketing exclusivity from the time of approval in the European Union (March 2014 through March 2024 in the case of bedaquiline).

EMA: European Medicines Agency; USG: United States government

[1] Lindsay McKenna, *The Price of Bedaquiline*, Treatment Action Group, 2018, http://www.treatmentactiongroup.org/sites/default/files/reality_check _bedaquiline_10_16_18.pdf.

INDEX

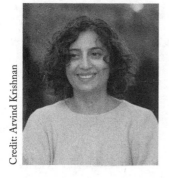

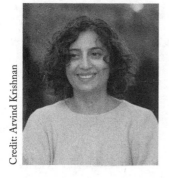Credit: Arvind Krishnan

Vidya Krishnan is an award-winning journalist who has been reporting on medical science for the last twenty years. She has written for the *Atlantic*, the *Los Angeles Times*, and the *Caravan*. She was a 2020–2021 Neiman Fellow at Harvard University.

PublicAffairs is a publishing house founded in 1997. It is a tribute to the standards, values, and flair of three persons who have served as mentors to countless reporters, writers, editors, and book people of all kinds, including me.

I. F. STONE, proprietor of *I. F. Stone's Weekly*, combined a commitment to the First Amendment with entrepreneurial zeal and reporting skill and became one of the great independent journalists in American history. At the age of eighty, Izzy published *The Trial of Socrates*, which was a national bestseller. He wrote the book after he taught himself ancient Greek.

BENJAMIN C. BRADLEE was for nearly thirty years the charismatic editorial leader of *The Washington Post*. It was Ben who gave the *Post* the range and courage to pursue such historic issues as Watergate. He supported his reporters with a tenacity that made them fearless and it is no accident that so many became authors of influential, best-selling books.

ROBERT L. BERNSTEIN, the chief executive of Random House for more than a quarter century, guided one of the nation's premier publishing houses. Bob was personally responsible for many books of political dissent and argument that challenged tyranny around the globe. He is also the founder and longtime chair of Human Rights Watch, one of the most respected human rights organizations in the world.

•　　•　　•

For fifty years, the banner of Public Affairs Press was carried by its owner Morris B. Schnapper, who published Gandhi, Nasser, Toynbee, Truman, and about 1,500 other authors. In 1983, Schnapper was described by *The Washington Post* as "a redoubtable gadfly." His legacy will endure in the books to come.

Peter Osnos, *Founder*

MAR 2 5 2022